The Food Alphabet
FOR HEART HEALTH

Learn your food ABCs and eat your way to awesome heart health!

Michelle Leon

DEDICATION

I would like to dedicate this book to my Grandfather Emile. He was a gentle and kind person that sadly suffered from heart problems later in life. My Grandad's lifestyle allowed him to live out most of his years healthy and strong and he saw the age of 93 that not many people get to see.

TABLE OF CONTENTS

ACKNOWLEDGMENTS

Firstly, I would like to thank Jehovah for giving me the strength and knowledge to write this book. Secondly, I would like to thank my family and friends who have supported me in all my endeavours over the years. I especially want to thank my mother who encouraged me to get writing and my sister-in-law Janine who suggested I write a book some years ago. Last but not least, I am grateful for my sister Melissa who took the courage to be the first writer in our family and helped the rest of us to take that step. Thank you to everyone who has supported me with this book!

CHAPTER 1

BACKGROUND

Hello reader! I hope this book finds you well. After reading, I hope that you will come away feeling more knowledgeable and confident about what to eat to prevent and even reverse heart disease.

The legend behind the book

Growing up, I always remember my grandfather being a very active man. One of his main hobbies was gardening and he often went with my grandma to a garden allotment. Unfortunately, gardening is not my strong point and I learnt that early on (when I somehow drowned the cress that I was trying to grow). However, I certainly was supportive of their hobby and was always keen to sample what they had grown!

Moving on, I also remember my Grandad having a healthy diet and fruit and nuts were always popular snacks when I went to visit him. I remember one time when my family visited St Lucia, my parents, along with my grandparents, went to visit my dad's aunt in the countryside. The house that my Great Auntie lived in was at the top of a steep hill. My Mother told me that in scorching heat, my 90-something-year-old grandfather seamlessly walked up this hill and even helped my Mum at times when she was struggling! I truly believe that his healthy lifestyle allowed him to have the quality of life he did, even when his health started to diminish in his early 90s. I say all this to emphasize that eating a healthy balanced diet as well as exercising and having a healthy lifestyle in general, won't guarantee old age, but it can certainly improve your quality of life, for however long you do live. My Grandad inspired me to write this book.

The Cardiovascular System

The cardiovascular system (also known as the circulatory system) is a crucial organ system and consists of the heart, blood vessels and blood. The heart acts as a pump forcing blood around the body.

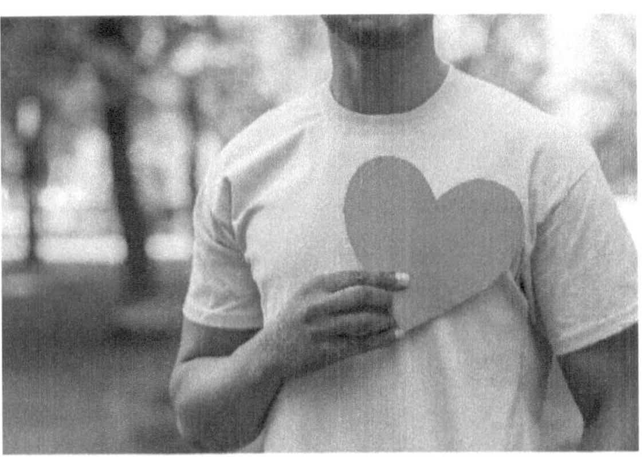

Within the cardiovascular system there are four types of blood vessels:

- **Arteries** are the elastic vessels that deliver oxygen-rich blood from the heart to the tissues of the body.

- **Veins**, in contrast to arteries, are elastic vessels that transport blood to the heart.

- **Capillaries** are extremely small vessels situated within the bodily tissues that transport blood from the arteries to the veins.

- **Sinusoids** are in the liver, spleen and bone marrow and are similar to capillaries but allow for much quicker nutrient absorption.

Heart disease

Heart disease (also known as cardiovascular disease) is a class of diseases that affect the heart and blood vessels (veins and arteries). According to the World Health Organization (WHO), heart disease still remains the leading cause of death worldwide (WHO, 2020). Heart disease is responsible for the loss of 18.6 million lives each year, which accounts for approximately 33% of all global deaths (NCD Alliance). Many types of conditions are classified under the heart disease umbrella, but the two biggest killers are coronary heart disease and ischaemic stroke (WHO, 2020). They are described as 'lifestyle diseases' because they are largely preventable (CDC, 2018). In fact, about 80% of premature deaths because of heart disease (between the ages of 30-70 years old) can be prevented.

Coronary heart disease (also known as coronary artery disease) is a serious condition where the arteries of the heart cannot deliver oxygen-rich blood to the heart due to a blood clot. Similarly, Ischaemic stroke is a serious condition where the blood flow in arteries that supply oxygen-rich blood to the brain is blocked due to a blood clot. Both conditions described are caused by a build-up of plaque in the arteries which causes the narrowing and hardening of the blood vessel. This, therefore, increases the risk of a blockage occurring when the blood passes through the artery. This phenomenon is called 'atherosclerosis'.

What we eat is critical to our health, especially for heart health. A person's risk of heart disease does have a genetic component as family history and ethnicity are linked to disease development (Williams et. al, 2015). However, many risk factors are modifiable and practising a healthy lifestyle provides a protective effect (CDC, 2018). Diet-related risk factors that increase the likelihood of developing heart disease include:

- Excess weight- being overweight, especially if you carry too much weight around your waist (NHS, 2022).

- High blood pressure (also known as hypertension)- High blood pressure that is consistently 140/90mmHg or higher will add to your risk (NHS, 2023). High blood pressure puts more strain on your heart and circulatory system. It places more added force against the artery walls.

- High cholesterol- Cholesterol is a fatty substance in your blood. We do need a small amount of blood cholesterol because the body uses it to build the structure of cell membranes, make hormones and helps our metabolism to work efficiently (Better Health Channel, 2022). However, too much cholesterol can increase your risk of heart disease.

- High blood sugar levels- when your blood sugar levels are consistently high, the body's ability to control your blood sugar levels by producing insulin (a hormone produced in the pancreas) diminishes. This is observed in pre-diabetes and uncontrolled Type 2 diabetes, which are both conditions largely linked to lifestyle practices (Diabetes UK). Having a high build of sugar in the blood can damage the arteries, making it more likely that atherosclerosis can occur (Diabetes UK).

- Metabolic Syndrome- this is the medical term for a combination of diabetes, high blood pressure (hypertension and stroke) and obesity. Metabolic syndrome affects an estimated 1 in 3 older adults aged 50 or over in the UK (NHS, 2022). As mentioned prior, all three conditions are risk factors, but having all three together will put you at a much greater risk of developing heart disease.

- Gum inflammation- Plaque is a sticky substance made from leftover food particles containing carbohydrates (sugars and starches) that mix with saliva in your mouth. A build of plaque along the gum line can lead to inflammation of the gums due to the many types of harmful bacteria found in plaque (Vera-Pineda et al. 2018). The bacteria can enter the bloodstream, promoting plaque formation and thus the progression of atherosclerosis.

Why read this book?

Not only can knowing what to eat help to prevent heart disease, but it can even reverse it as healing of the arteries can take place (Williams et al., 2015). Arteries, which are the blood vessels that deliver oxygen-rich blood from the heart to the tissues of the body, have been shown by medical research to have the potential to heal (Williams et al., 2015).

If you practice a healthy balanced diet, you will already be doing yourself a huge favour in regard to heart health. General healthy eating guides and models are listed below:

- The Eatwell Guide (UK)

- Canada's Food Guide

- My Plate (USA)

However, some foods have been identified as particularly beneficial to heart health and have been labelled as 'cardio-protective'. The term cardio-protective describes entities that serve to protect the heart or arteries from injury, disease, or malfunction [5].

Not all foods are created equal and although some foods have been identified as cardio-protective in nature, it doesn't mean it has been well researched and the strength of evidence supporting its beneficial effects on heart health is strong.

For this reason, at the end of the book, I will be presenting a **food alphabet for heart health checklist for you to** implement into your dietary practices. I will take you on a journey discussing foods argued to have cardio-protective properties and at the end, present the foods that qualified for the credible food alphabet for heart health checklist. To make the list, certain criteria had to be met for a particular food to be selected.

The criteria to make the checklist were deliberately strict and the food item had to meet at least three of the following standards:

- The food item had to be well-researched.
- The food item had to be a whole food i.e., unprocessed or unrefined with the exception of a food item being drained or cooked for safety purposes.
- The evidence on the heart health benefits of the food item had to be from the highest forms of evidence (level 1). These currently are systematic reviews and meta-analyses. For more information about these types of research, please have a look at this website:

- The findings around the heart health benefits of the food items had to be consistent.

Often you can get health professionals telling you to eat certain foods, but there isn't much information on why they are helpful. Therefore, this book will explain why these foods are so special and you will provide you with 'Top Tips' on how each food item could be added to your diet. In addition, you will also find several tasty recipes along the way & other resources as a bonus.

Please note that it is not possible to provide a list of cardio-protective foods for <u>each letter of the alphabet</u>. Only foods that have been identified as having a link to heart health are included.

CHAPTER 2

HOW HEALTHY IS YOUR DIET? QUIZ

Before we delve into discussing different cardio-protective foods, the backbone of a good diet for heart health (as mentioned in the previous chapter) is a healthy diet. Therefore, I have created a very simple healthy eating quiz to help you gauge how healthy your diet is currently. We can all improve our diets in some way, so the aim is not necessarily to get a perfect score straight away.

There is a total of 30 points depending on your question response. The responses to the questions are of a multiple-choice style and are based on the British Eat-well guide. In the multiple-choice selections, all choices will be marked with a number that represents how many points the response is worth.

There is a traffic light system to interpret your score.

GREEN= Small improvements to diet required
AMBER= Moderate improvements to diet required
RED=Large improvements to diet required

HEALTHY EATING QUIZ

Eating habits

1. **Do you go for long periods without eating during the day? (a gap of 4 hours or more)**

   A.   Yes (2)
   B.   No (0)

2. **Do you have 3 main meals during the day (breakfast, lunch, and dinner)?**

   A.   Yes (1)
   B.   No (0)

Adults are recommended to eat regularly throughout the day.

Fluids

3. **Do you drink mainly unsweetened drinks during the day?**

   C.   Yes (1)
   D.   No (0)

4. **Do you drink water throughout the day?**

   A.   Yes (2)
   B.   No (0)

Adults are recommended to have 6-8 glasses of fluid a day.

Fruit and vegetables

5. Do you eat at least 5 fruit and vegetables a day?

    E.   Yes (2)
    F.   No (0)

6. Do you eat a variety of different fruit and vegetables?

    A.   Yes (1)
    B.   No (0)

Adults are recommended to have at least 5 portions of dairy a day.

Dairy foods (includes animal or plant-based milk, cheese, yoghurt etc.) For portion size, use a cup of milk, a matchbox size of cheese and a pot of yoghurt as a reference.

7. Do you have at least one portion of dairy a day?

    G.   Yes (1)
    H.   No (0)

8. Do you have 2-3 portions of dairy a day?

    A.   Yes (2)
    B.   No (0)

Adults are recommended to have 2-3 portions of dairy a day.

Starchy carbohydrates (e.g., rice, potato, pasta, cous cous, buckwheat, quinoa etc.)

9. **Do you eat at least 3 different starchy foods a day?**

    I. **Yes (2)**
    J. **No (0)**

10. **Do you regularly eat wholegrain versions? (e.g., wholegrain pasta, rice etc.)**

    A. **Yes (1)**
    B. **No (0)**

Adults are recommended to have 3-4 portions of starchy carbohydrates a day.

Protein (includes animal or plant protein sources such as legumes, eggs, nuts, fish, chicken, beef etc.) For portion size, use the palm of your hand as a reference.

11. **Do you have at least one portion of protein a day?**

    K. **Yes (1)**
    L. **No (0)**

12. **Do you have 2-3 portions of protein a day?**

    A. **Yes (2)**
    B. **No (0)**

Adults are recommended to have 2-3 portions of protein a day.

Salt and sugar intake

13. Do you add salt and sugar to your food regularly?

    M.   Yes (2)
    N.   No (0)

14. Do you limit your intake of processed foods daily? (Foods high in fat, salt and sugar such as chocolate, bacon, crisps, biscuits etc.)

    A.   Yes (1)
    B.   No (0)

Adults are recommended to limit the amount of added sugar and salt consumed over the day.

Shopping habits

15. Do you choose low-fat products when available? (e.g., reduced fat mince, yoghurt etc.)

    O.   Yes (1)
    P.   No (0)

16. Do you limit purchasing foods high in salt, fat and sugar?

    A.   Yes (2)
    B.   No (0)

Adults are recommended to read the traffic light labels to help them determine the nutrition of products they buy.

Cooking habits

17. **Do you mostly bake, steam or grill instead of frying foods?**

    Q.   **Yes (2)**
    R.   **No (0)**

18. **Do you minimize the amount of salt and sugar you use in recipes?**
19.

    A.   **Yes (1)**
    B.   **No (0)**

Adults are recommended to limit their saturated fat, salt and sugar intake.

Alcohol intake

20. **Do you drink no more than 14 units of alcohol a week?** As a reference, a unit of alcohol is a single shot of spirit.

    S.   **Yes (1)**
    T.   **No (0)**

21. **Do you space out your alcoholic drinks?**

    A.   **Yes (2)**
    B.   **No (0)**

Adults are recommended to have no more than 14 units of alcohol a week and not binge drink (having multiple alcoholic drinks in one go)

You have come to the end of the quiz!

Scoring table

Question	Points
1	/2
2	/1
3	/1
4	/2
5	/2
6	/1
7	/1
8	/2
9	/2
10	/1
11	/1
12	/2
13	/2
14	/1
15	/1
16	/2
17	/2
18	/1
19	/1
20	/2
Total:	/30

GREEN (21-30) = Small improvements required
AMBER (11-20) = Moderate improvements required
RED (0-10) =Large improvements required

Tick or circle the categories below, where you feel positive changes can be made.

- **Eating habits**
- **Fluids**
- **Fruit and vegetables**
- **Dairy foods**
- **Carbohydrate**
- **Protein**
- **Salt and sugar intake**
- **Shopping habits**
- **Cooking method**
- **Alcohol intake**

Next, we will start our journey by looking at different foods that have been reported to have cardio-protective properties. What will make the ultimate food alphabet for heart health checklist? Read to the end to find out.

CHAPTER 3

A IS FOR ALMONDS

What are Almonds?

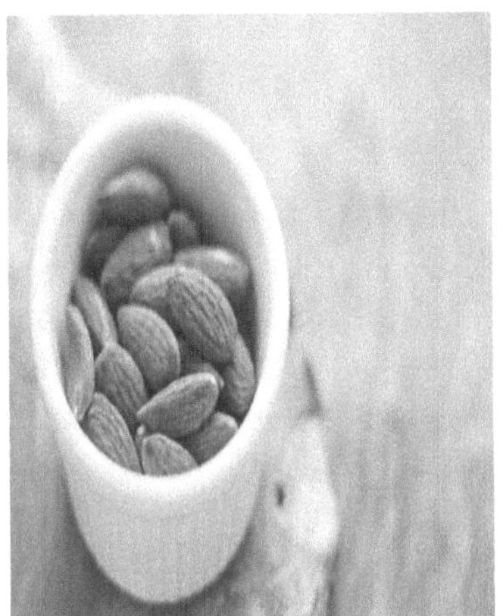

Almonds most commonly referred to as a nut, are actually edible seeds of the Almond Tree. The Almond tree is a species of tree native to Iran and the Middle East, but almonds are cultivated globally, with the US being the largest producer. There are two types of almonds- bitter or sweet. Bitter almonds are inedible and are used to make almond oil.

Why is it good for heart health?

Almonds are packed with nutrients and vitamin E, fibre calcium, iron, riboflavin, and magnesium. Almonds are considered to be especially good for the heart because they are a rich source of healthy fats (mono- and polyunsaturated fatty acids), which have been shown to have positive effects on low-density lipoprotein (LDL) and high-density lipoprotein (HDL) (Feingold et al., 2018). LDL is known as the 'bad' cholesterol and HDL is known as the 'good' cholesterol. So, let's delve further into what LDL and HDL are.

A lipoprotein is a complex molecule made up of many proteins. The function of lipoproteins is to transport cholesterol (fat molecules) around the body (de Souza et al., 2017). HDL is known as the 'good' cholesterol because it acts like a scavenger and picks up cholesterol in your blood and transports it to your liver, where any excess fat can be expelled from the body. Contrastingly, LDL is known as bad cholesterol, because it takes cholesterol to your arteries where it may build up in your arteries. Too much fat in your arteries leads to a build-up of fatty plaque called atherosclerosis.

The addition of almonds to the diet has been shown to decrease LDL and maintain HDL (Feingold et al., 2018). This means that eating almonds could help to reduce any unhealthy levels of fat in the arteries and prevent the development or worsening of atherosclerosis (Eslami et., 2019).

Top tips!

Due to the high energy density of nuts and seeds, it was believed that their consumption could increase weight gain; however, it is observed that the consumption of this group of foods does not stimulate weight gain **when eaten whole** (Hollingworth et al., 2019). Therefore, if you are trying to avoid weight gain, limit your use of nuts and seed butter. Avoid nuts and seeds coated in sugar, chocolate, salt, or honey-roasted varieties.

- Having a handful of raw almonds (about 30 grams) a day makes a pretty good snack! Due to the high fibre content of almonds, consumption makes you feel fuller for longer[10]. Please note that due to the high fibre content, excessive consumption may cause constipation.

- Sprinkle some almonds onto your cereal for a lovely, tasty addition!

- Add to a seasonal green salad for extra crunch.

- To add flavour to almonds in a healthy way, spray almonds lightly with vegetable oil spray on a baking tray. Then experiment with different spices and herbs. For spicy almonds, sprinkle cayenne, garlic, chilli, and cumin powder. Bake the almonds at 200 degrees Celsius (180 if fan assisted) for 15 minutes. After fully cooling store in a Ziploc freezer bag or airtight container. Black pepper and lemon are also good flavours.

CHAPTER 4

B IS FOR BEETROOT AND BERRIES

What is Beetroot?

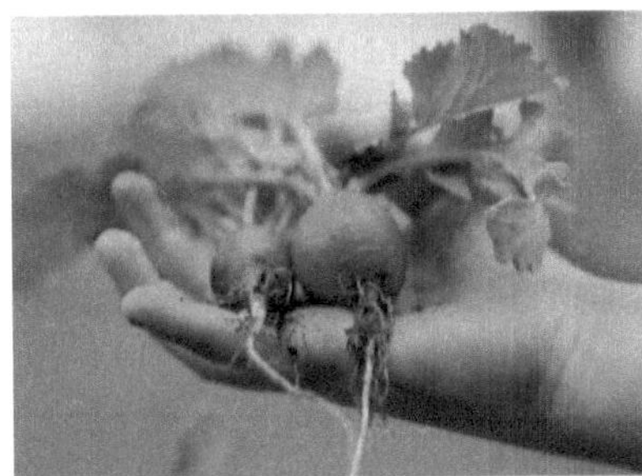

Beetroot (also known as beet) is a portion of the beet plant and is consumed as a root vegetable. The most common type is red beetroot, which has dark pink/purple flesh and an earthy, rich flavour.

Why is it good for heart health?

There is strong evidence that a diet high in fruit and vegetables is protective against cardiovascular disease (Bonilla et al. 2018). Fruit and vegetables are full of many nutrients and compounds that are beneficial to heart health. Beetroot has been identified as a vegetable that is particularly cardio-protective (Saman et al. 2015). Beetroot contains nitrates which have a positive effect on a chemical called 'nitric oxide'. This chemical helps to widen the blood vessels by dilation, allowing more blood to go through the vessel at reduced pressure. Therefore, beetroot is effective in reducing blood pressure (Saman et al. 2015).

When you have blood passing through at high pressure, it is more likely to cause damage to the blood vessels. The force of the blood could break off any plaque build-up (i.e., atherosclerotic lesions) and if the blood vessels are narrow; this is more likely to cause a blockage. This can lead to a heart attack or stroke, as oxygenated blood is cut off from the heart or brain due to the blockage.

Top tips!

- In line with general government guidance, aim to eat at least five fruit and vegetables a day for health benefits.

- Try drinking a cup of raw unsweetened beetroot juice (approx. 250ml) daily.

- You can also consider adding beetroot as an accompaniment for many dishes such as salads, roasts, soups, noodles, pasta etc.

What are berries?

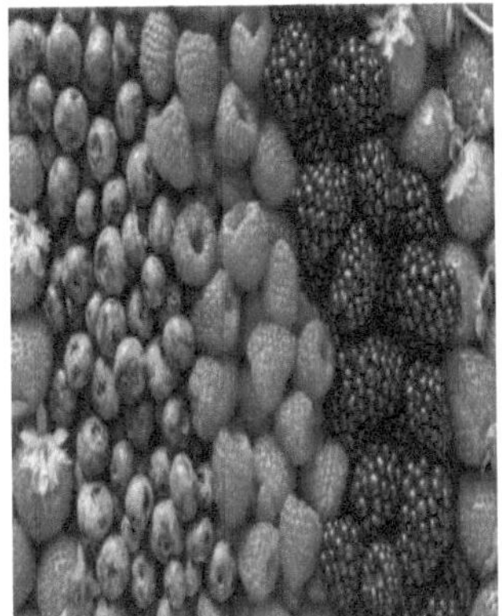 A berry is a soft fleshy fruit that is without a stone (pit) and contains little seeds. Most people are familiar with the common berries sold in shops such as blueberries, strawberries, blackberries, and raspberries. However, there are around 27 different types of berries.

Why is it good for heart health?

As mentioned previously, there is strong evidence that a diet high in fruit and vegetables is protective against cardiovascular disease (Bonilla et al. 2018). Fruit and vegetables are full of many nutrients and compounds that are beneficial to heart health (Bonilla et al. 2018). Berries are a good source of polyphenols and due to this, have been identified by human intervention studies to be particularly cardio-protective (Luís et al., 2018).

Polyphenols are a type of antioxidant that protects plants from UV rays and attacks from pathogens and have now been recognized as also being beneficial to human health (Charis et al. 2021). Antioxidants are molecules that inhibit oxidation, a process whereby oxygen is added to a compound and due to this interaction, an unstable molecule called a 'free radical' is formed. Free radicals in the environment damage cells. An imbalance of free radicals and antioxidants in the body leads to a state of what is called 'oxidative stress'. In this situation, the body is unable to effectively prevent free radical damage to cells.

In heart health, polyphenols protect LDL molecules (the 'bad' cholesterol) from becoming unstable by interactions with free radicals (Potì et al., 2019). When LDL molecules become unstable, by a process called oxidation, this cholesterol can become more reactive with the lining of blood vessels and promote atherosclerosis.

Top tips!

- In line with general government guidance, try to eat at least five fruit and vegetables a day for health benefits.

- Having a handful of blueberries (about 80 grams) a day makes a pretty good snack! This will count towards your 5 a day.

- Sprinkle some blueberries onto your cereal for a lovely, tasty addition!

- Add them to a vegetable smoothie for sweetness.

Recipe 2

Spruce your breakfast up by trying these overnight oats!

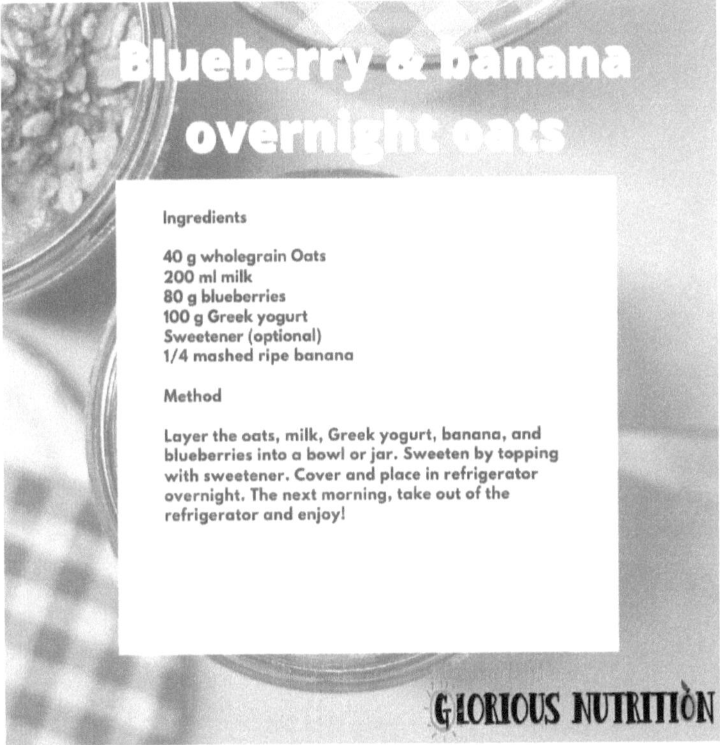

CHAPTER 5

C IS FOR CINNAMON

What is cinnamon?

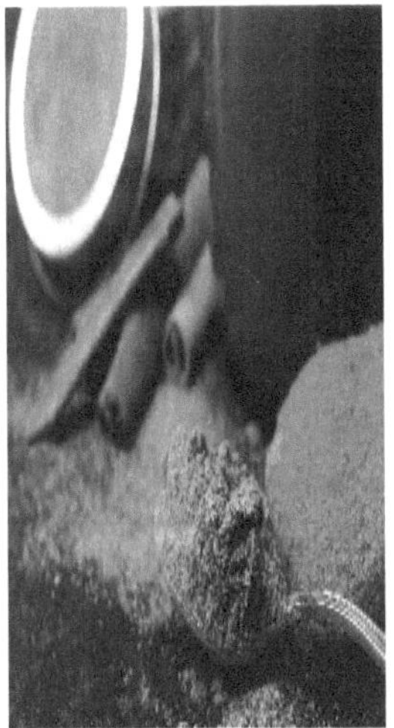

Cinnamon is an aromatic spice made from the peeled, dried, and rolled bark of two tropical trees in Asia called Cinnamomum cassia (from Southern China) and Southeast Asia, Cinnamomum verum/C. verum (formerly C. zeylanicum). The C. verum tree is generally called the "true cinnamon tree" or "Ceylon cinnamon tree". Cinnamon is a popular spice that is used in many cuisines and beverages for its distinctive aroma and taste. Essential oils made from cinnamon are also widely used in the food and cosmetic industries.

Why is it good for heart health?

Cinnamon can prevent high blood pressure and reduce LDL cholesterol, which are both linked to the development of heart disease (Mollazedah et al. 2016).

Cinnamon is packed with polyphenols, which as mentioned in previous chapters are plant compounds with protective antioxidant properties that inhibit damage to cells from free radical activity. Due to this, the consumption of cinnamon helps to prevent damage to arteries from LDL-cholesterol molecules because of interaction with free radicals.

In addition, the compound called cinnamaldehyde which gives cinnamon its odour and flavour, can support the dilation of the arteries (vasorelaxation), resulting in a reduction in blood pressure.

Moreover, cinnamon consumption has been found to reduce blood cholesterol and in particular LDL cholesterol (Askari et., 2014) (Khan et al., 2003). For instance, one study found that intake of 1, 3, or 6 g of cinnamon per day reduced serum glucose, triglyceride, LDL cholesterol, and total cholesterol (Khan et al. 2003).

Top tips!

- Cinnamon is naturally sweet, so you can sprinkle it on your porridge, or toast.

- The sweet spice also works well with savoury dishes such as curries and soups.

- Dust plain nuts with cinnamon powder and roast in the oven.

- You can add cinnamon to drinks as a natural sweetener. E.g., you can add it to a vegetable and fruit smoothie or plain milk.

- Make cinnamon tea by:

  o Breaking up a cinnamon stick and add it to water in a pot.
  o Bring the water to a boil and simmer for 2-3 minutes.
  o Strain the tea into a cup and allow it to cool for one minute before drinking.

- Cinnamon contains coumarin, a compound that can be harmful to the liver in large amounts (European Food Safety Authority, 2004). Coumarin levels are higher in Cassia cinnamon than in Ceylon cinnamon.

Therefore, if you are unsure about what cinnamon you are using, it is recommended to only have up to 1 teaspoon of cinnamon a day (as this is the safe limit for Cassia cinnamon). This would equate to roughly using cinnamon **once per day**.

- Using cinnamon bark or powder is better but if you don't like the taste, you can consider taking supplements. Avoid taking cinnamon supplements if you are pregnant or under 18 years of age as the safety of cinnamon supplementation is unknown. Also, if you are on any medications, especially ones that affect the liver, it is recommended to seek medical advice before deciding.

CHAPTER 6

D IS FOR DAIRY AND DARK CHOCOLATE

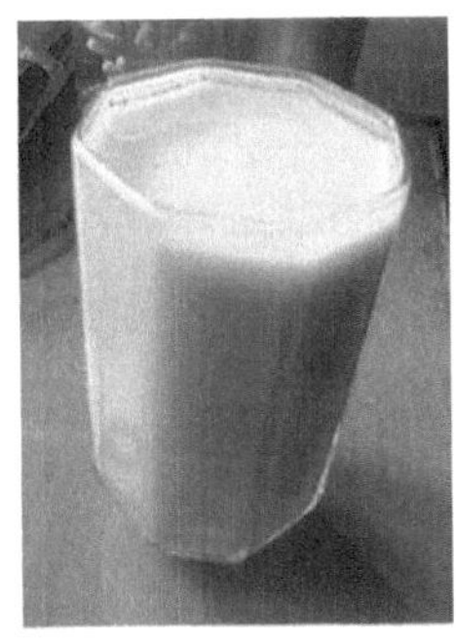

What are dairy foods?

Dairy is a food group and consists of foods made from the milk of mammals (such as cows, buffalo, goats etc.) or plant-based milk (e.g., almond, soya, cashew etc.). Dairy foods include milk, yoghurt and cheese, butter, and cream.

Why is it good for heart health?

Dairy is a nutritious food that can be part of a heart-healthy dietary pattern. Dairy products contain a matrix of nutrients such as vitamins and minerals (such as calcium and vitamin D), amino acids (the building blocks of proteins) and fatty acids (the building blocks of fats). The more processed a dairy product is, the less array of nutrients it will have. The complementary working of individual nutrients within dairy as a whole, rather than single nutrients is believed to be what makes dairy beneficial to heart health (Anand et al. 2015). The benefits to heart health are the following (Anand et al. 2015):

- Blood pressure management
- Improvement in the blood lipid profile
- An increase in insulin sensitivity- Insulin is a hormone that helps us to control our blood sugar levels. It is produced by the pancreas. Too much sugar in the blood on a consistent basis can damage the blood vessels.
- Weight management benefit- due to benefits to appetite control and the breakdown of fat in the body.

Dairy foods that have been fermented with lactic acid bacteria such as Lactobacillus have been particularly reported to reduce the risk of heart disease (Tholstrup et al. 2006) (Anand et al. 2015). Examples include kefir and yoghurt. Fermented foods can contain 'probiotics' – live bacteria and yeasts that are thought to have health benefits.

Top tips!

- Choose unsweetened versions of dairy products.

- It is important if choosing plant milk to make sure that it says on the label that it is fortified, especially with calcium. Non-fortified plant milk has minimal nutritional value.

- Predominantly choose low-fat dairy products.

- Butter is high in fat and saturated fat. It can often be high in salt, too, so try to eat it less often and in small amounts.

- Cream is also high in fat, so use this less often and in small amounts, too. You can use lower-fat plain yoghurt and fromage frais instead of cream.

- Some cheeses can also be high in salt. More than 1.5g salt per 100g is considered high.

What is Dark chocolate?

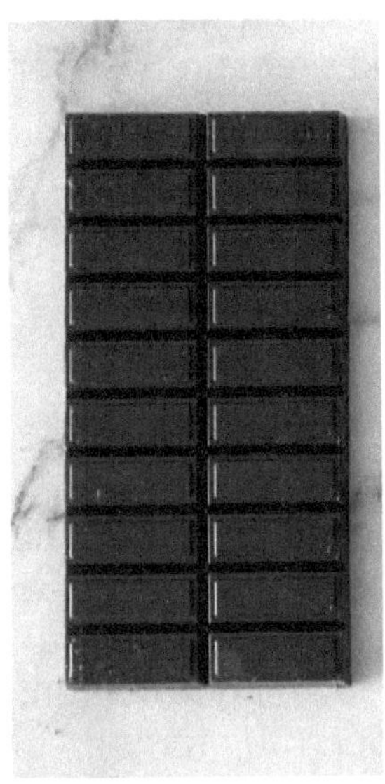

Dark chocolate is a bitter-tasting food in the form of a paste or solid block made mostly from processed cocoa butter and solids. Cocoa is a brown powder made from the roasted seeds (cocoa beans) of the cocoa tree. Dark chocolate contains the highest amount of cocoa than any other type of chocolate. In fact, dark chocolate contains 50-90% cocoa solids and cocoa butter, whereas milk chocolate only contains approximately anywhere from 10-20%. Dark chocolate should contain no milk (unless there is cross-contamination during processing) and a small amount of sugar.

Why is it good for heart health?

Dark chocolate is rich in minerals, such as iron, magnesium, and zinc which are all beneficial to heart health. However, the functional ingredient in dark chocolate that has been argued to be largely responsible for a positive impact on heart health is cocoa. Cocoa is a rich source of compounds called flavonoids (a type of polyphenol) which has both anti-inflammatory and antioxidant properties. One type of flavanol in particular that has been researched regarding the effects of dark chocolate and heart health is epicatechin. Most manufacturers don't include flavanol content on their labels but approximately 20g of dark chocolate (60% cocoa solids) contains 34mg of flavanols (Dm coffee blog, 2022).

The flavanols in dark chocolate are believed to stimulate the endothelium (the lining of the arteries), to produce nitric oxide (NO). As mentioned previously, nitric oxide is required by the arteries to dilate and when the blood vessels dilate, blood pressure decreases. Some controlled studies show that cocoa and dark chocolate have a mild but positive impact improve blood flow and lower blood pressure (Fisher et al., 2002) (Faridi 2008), (Shiini 2009) (Heiss et al., 2007).

Top tips!

- Make sure to read the food labels of dark chocolate products. When looking for dark chocolate:
    - Look for bars with a cocoa content of 70% or higher. A higher percentage of cocoa means a higher number of flavonoids.
    - Choose dark chocolate with low sugar content (less than 5 grams of sugar per 100 grams).

- Aim to consume 1-2 bars (20-30grams) of dark chocolate regularly.

CHAPTER 7

E IS FOR EGGPLANT

What is Eggplant?

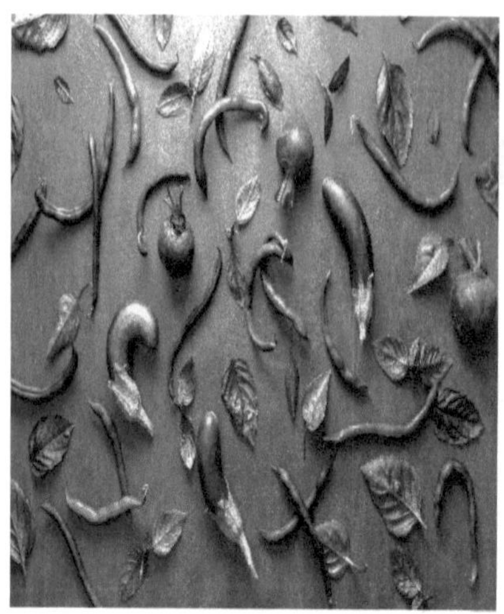

Eggplant (Solanum melongea) is a tender perennial plant species in the nightshade family Solanaceae. Eggplant is also known as aubergine, brinjal and 'Guinea squash'. Although technically a fruit, eggplant is consumed as a vegetable and is spongey in texture. It is available in different colours and shapes, but the tear-shaped purple variety commonly is the one most sold in shops.

Why is it good for heart health?

Eggplant has been identified as possessing antioxidant properties that may help to support heart health (Scorsatto et al. 2019). For instance, the vegetable contains the polyphenol antioxidant called Nasunin which has been particularly investigated in relation to heart health (Das et al. 2011). Eggplant has been found to increase the antioxidant capacity in the blood (Scorsatto et al. 2019). This would suggest that eggplant consumption could be beneficial in helping the body to fight against free radicals that attempt to damage the arteries and other cells in the body in the absence of sufficient antioxidant concentrations.

Additionally, eggplant is rich in dietary fibre and has the potential to positively impact the blood cholesterol profile. (Yarmohammadi et al. 2021) Preventing high blood cholesterol is likely to reduce the risk of developing heart disease. For example, a study by Guimarãe et al. 2000 found that in a group of 38 patients with high blood cholesterol, after 5 weeks, eggplant had a modest, positive effect on their blood cholesterol profiles.

Top tips!

- Eggplant is a versatile vegetable and can easily be incorporated as one of your 5 a day.

- Aside from the green top, everything else from the eggplant is entirely edible (skin, white flesh, seeds). If your eggplant is young and tender, the nutrient skin-skin will be less tough and is perfect for skillet frying or braising with a little oil.

- Eggplant can be added to curries or a lamb (or vegetable) tagine. Just cut into cubes, add to the sauce, and cook until tender. Serve with brown rice.

- You could roast eggplant and serve it with pasta.

- Try adding eggplant to a stir-fry. To ensure it cooks thoroughly, add it to the stir-fry early.

- Instead of pasta sheets, you can use eggplant to make lasagne. To do this slice the vegetable lengthwise into thin sheets.

- You can use eggplant to make ratatouille (stewed vegetables). Serve with crusty brown or sourdough bread.

- You can add eggplant as an extra topping on homemade pizza.

CHAPTER 8

F IS FOR FLAXSEED

What is Flaxseed?

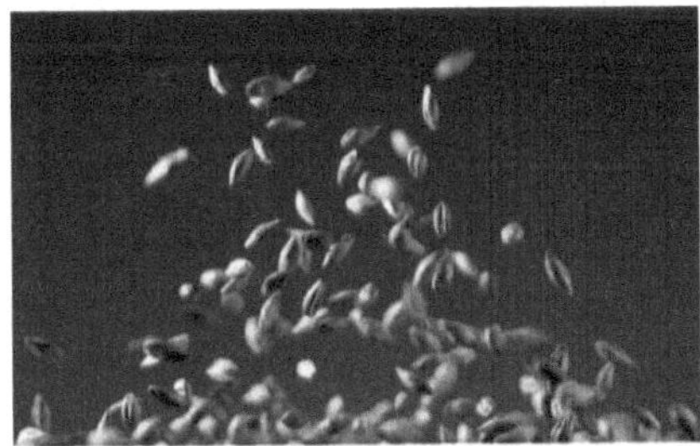

Flaxseed also known as linseed, is a small seed that comes from the flax plant. This is cultivated in cooler regions of the world.

Why is it good for heart health?

Flaxseed has been found to significantly reduce blood pressure by positively impacting blood cholesterol levels (Sorin et al., 2016). Flaxseed contains a range of powerful compounds that allow this cardio-protective effect to take place. To begin, flaxseeds are a rich source of ALA (alpha-linolenic acid), an essential omega-3 fatty acid that is a healthy dietary fat (Obermeyer et al. 1995). Due to the presence of ALA, the consumption of flaxseed has been found to lead to an increase in HDL, the 'good' cholesterol (that helps excess fat in the body to be expelled) (Sorin et al., 2016). In addition, flaxseeds are one of the best sources of:

- Phytoestrogens (lignans)
- Phytosterols
- Dietary fibre

Never heard of phytoestrogens? Well, this is a plant compound that has a similar structure to human oestrogen. Phytoestrogens protect the blood from free radicals (unstable molecules) that inhibit the ability of arteries to dilate properly (Ried et al., 2008). Free radicals interfere with the presence of nitric oxide. As mentioned previously, nitric oxide is required by the arteries to dilate and when the blood vessels dilate, blood pressure decreases.

Then we have phytosterols. Never heard of this either? Well, this is also a plant compound that amazingly has a similar structure to cholesterol. When digested, they compete with cholesterol absorption in our intestines, so that less cholesterol is absorbed into the bloodstream.

Last but not least, we have fibre, an often-unsung health hero. Fibre interferes with cholesterol absorption by binding to cholesterol particles during the digestion process. This causes less cholesterol to enter the bloodstream.

Top tips!

- Consider using flaxseed for at least 3 months to see significant benefits.

- Make a habit of adding a tablespoon of grounded flaxseed to bread, soups, cereals, yoghurts, salads, smoothies, porridge and pretty much anything that takes your fancy!

- Consider using flaxseed for at least 3 months to see significant benefits.

- Make a habit of adding a tablespoon of grounded flaxseed to bread, soups, cereals, yoghurts, salads, smoothies, porridge and pretty much anything that takes your fancy!

Recipe time!

Homemade Flaxseed Crackers

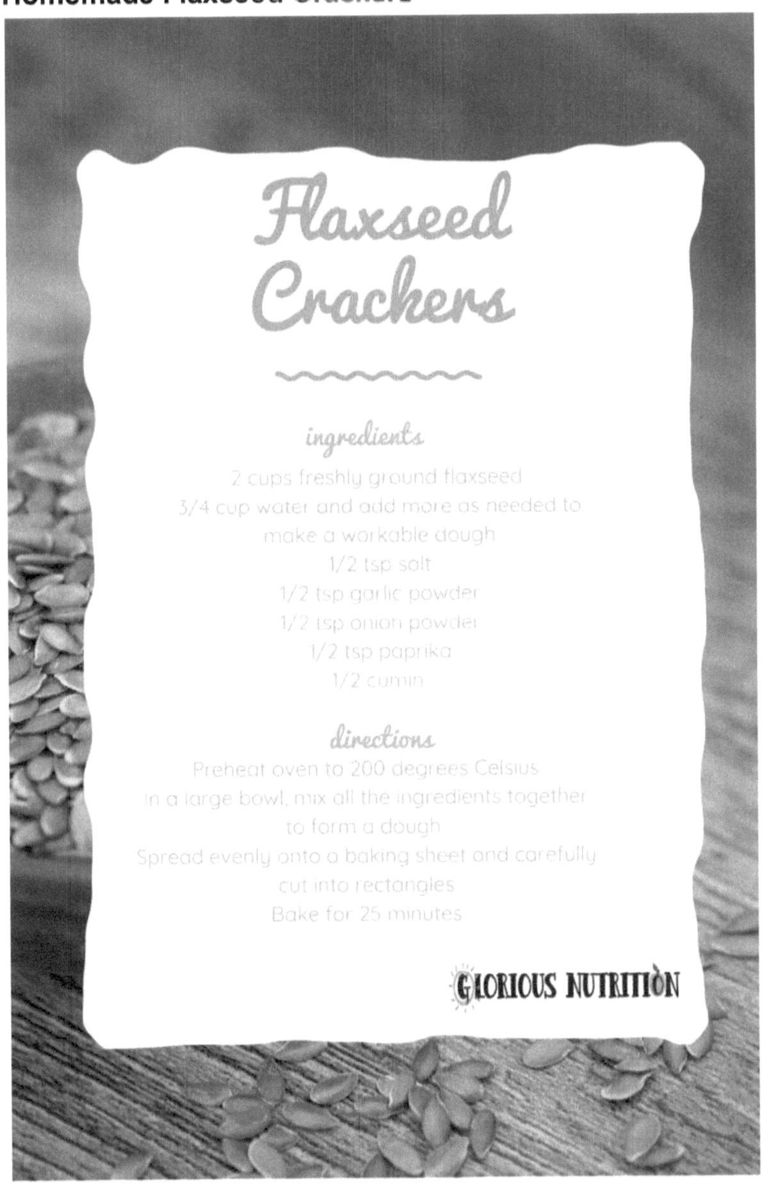

CHAPTER 9

G IS FOR GARLIC

What is Garlic?

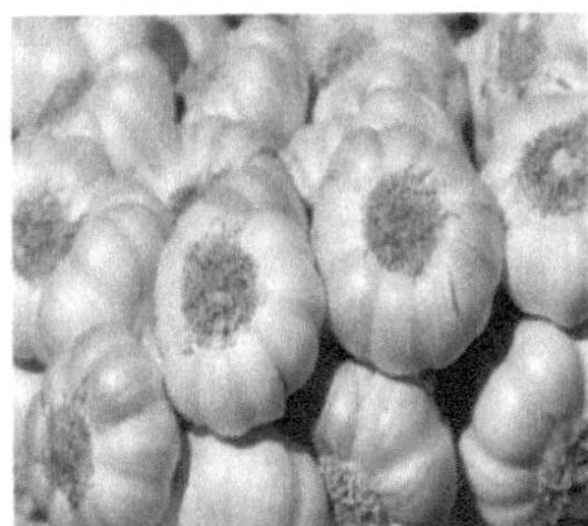 Garlic is a plant that is a close relative to onions, shallots, and leeks. The garlic cloves taken from the garlic bulb are used as a vegetable. Garlic originates from Central Asia and North-Eastern Iran.

Why is it good for heart health?

For centuries, garlic has been widely used to support heart health. Garlic contains nutrients such as vitamin C, manganese, vitamin B6, and selenium. Also, garlic contains a chemical called allicin, a type of antioxidant containing sulphur compounds, which is thought to be responsible for its positive effects on heart health (Reid et al. 2008). Allicin is an oily, slightly yellow liquid that is responsible for the distinctive odour of raw garlic. Research has found garlic consumption to be attributable to significant reductions in blood pressure (Reid et al. 2014). The mechanism believed to be responsible for this beneficial reduction in blood pressure due to garlic consumption, is the ability of the presence of allicin to increase the body's production of nitric oxide (Reid et al. 2014). As mentioned in Chapter 4, nitric oxide is required by the arteries to dilate; when the blood vessels dilate, blood pressure decreases. Garlic has also been found to reduce total blood cholesterol (Aslani et al. 2016).

Adding lemon to a garlic mixture is anecdotally cited as a traditional natural remedy to prevent and treat high blood pressure. Lemon is high in potassium which is good for blood pressure. It is also high in erycosytryn and hesperidin flavones which have been found in animal studies to decrease oxidative stress which would be beneficial to heart health. However, no evidence was identified to suggest that lemon **on its own** has a cardioprotective effect in humans. In contrast, there is evidence to support that combining garlic with lemon does have an observed positive effect on heart health. For instance, a study by (Aslani et al. 2016) found ingestion of a garlic and lemon juice mixture after 8 weeks led to an improvement in cardiovascular risk factors. This included a reduction in total blood cholesterol, blood pressure, body mass index and fibrinogen (a compound that rises in response to systemic inflammation and tissue injury) (Aslani et al. 2016).

Top tips!

- There is no reference nutrient intake (RNI) for garlic. However, it's safe to consume at normal levels found in your food (about 1-2 cloves).

- Some people may be allergic to garlic, so if you experience any unpleasant side effects stop consuming it and seek the advice of your GP.

- Mince 2-3 garlic cloves and add to soups, salads, and one-pot dishes like shepherd's pie.

- Add a clove of garlic to herbal teas.

- Try making your garlic butter by mincing garlic with olive spread. The butter can then be added to bread or jacket potato. Why not make your own garlic bread? It is recommended to use wholemeal, wholegrain, or seeded bread over white bread, if possible, due to the higher fibre content.

- Try to stick to fresh garlic as some evidence suggests that ready-chopped garlic that is stored in oil or water, and odourless garlic products have lower allicin levels.

- Add 1 or 2 garlic cloves to a vegetable smoothie and use 150ml of fruit juice for sweetness.

- Make your own salad dressing by mincing garlic and adding it to extra virgin olive oil with a splash of lemon.

- Garlic supplements can be used but please read the label before use and seek medical advice if you are unsure. Be careful of contraindications with other medicines e.g., garlic supplements can interfere with anti-coagulation or anti-platelet medications.

Recipe time!

As well as using garlic to add flavour to meals, why not try garlic tea? Check out this garlic tea recipe!

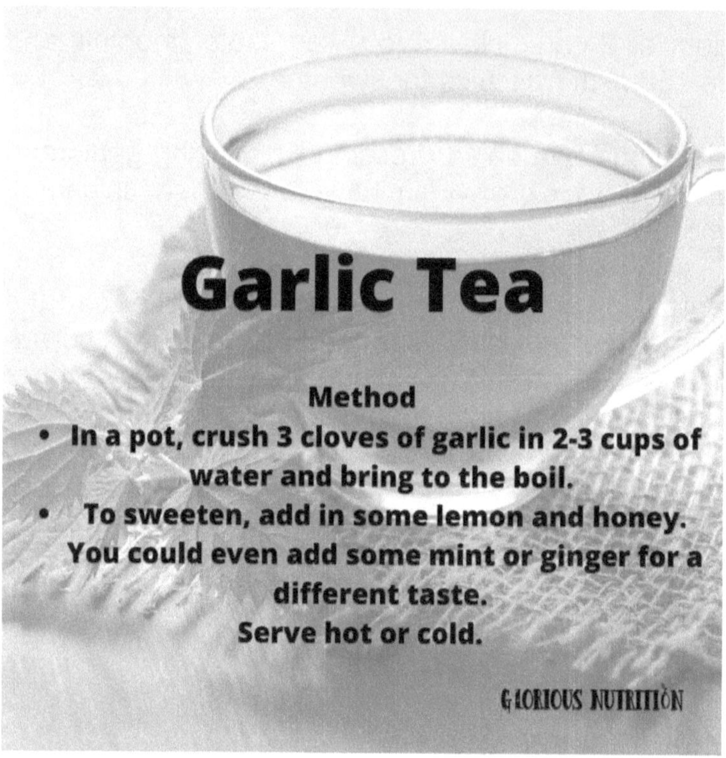

CHAPTER 10

K IS FOR KALE

What is Kale?

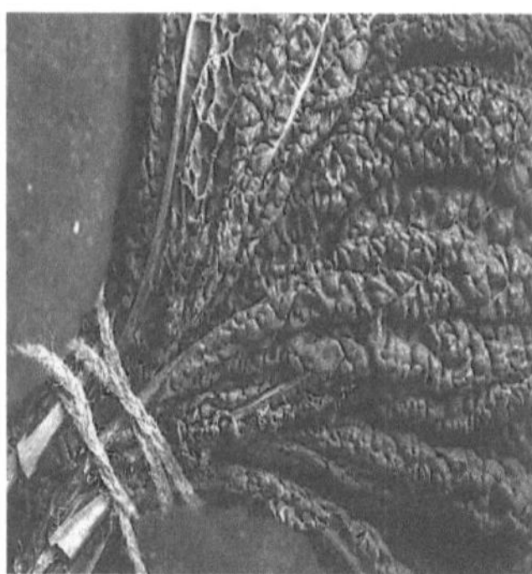 Kale (also known as leaf cabbage) is a green leafy cruciferous vegetable that belongs to the cabbage family. It was originally known as 'cole' or 'colewort' in England but now most people call it by its Scottish name, kale (BBC Good Food).

Why is it good for heart health?

One serving of kale provides at least 10% of the recommended daily allowance for 17 essential nutrients. Due to this, kale has been stated to be a 'powerhouse food' according to a Centres for Disease Control study of fruit and vegetables (Noia et al., 2014). The bioactive component believed to give kale and other green leafy vegetables their cardioprotective properties is the presence of nitrates in this vegetable type. As mentioned before in Chapter 4, nitrates are compounds that widen the blood vessels through dilation, allowing more blood to travel through the blood vessel at reduced pressure. Therefore, consuming green leafy vegetables such as kale that are high in nitrates can help to reduce blood pressure, a common risk factor for heart disease.

Meta-analyses (whereby multiple study results are pooled together) have found that green leafy vegetable intake was associated with a reduced incidence of heart disease (Pollock, 2016), (Ojagbemi et al., 2021).

Moreover, one study found that one cup of raw (or half a cup of cooked) leafy green vegetables each day, can significantly reduce a person's risk of heart disease (Science Daily,

2021). Another study that looked at kale in particular, found that 3-month kale juice supplementation in men with high blood cholesterol, increased blood antioxidant activity and reduced total blood cholesterol; which both will reduce heart disease risk (Kim et.al, 2008).

Top tips!
- Kale can be quite tough, so it is best parboiled before being fried, or steamed for 5-10 minutes.

- Make a leafy green vegetable smoothie and use 150ml of fruit juice for sweetness. You could even add some Greek yoghurt for a creamy texture.

- Try making your own pesto with spinach, broccoli or kale.

- Kale can be a great addition to sauces, soups and salads.

- Make a tasty omelette or baked eggs with chopped kale.

- Add to a pasta bake.

CHAPTER 11

L IS FOR LEGUMES

What are Legumes?

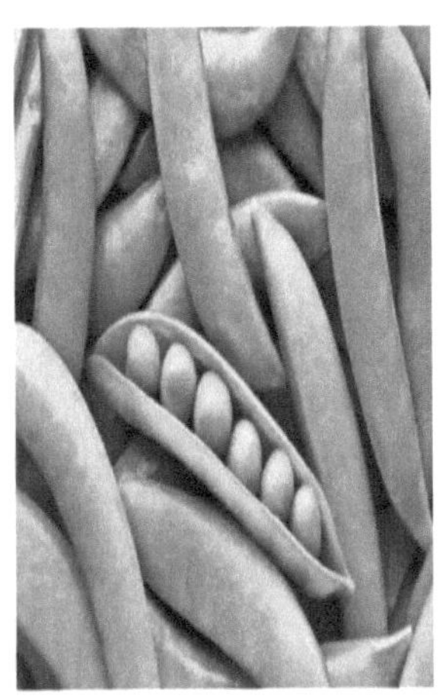

A legume is a plant belonging to the plant family Fabaceae and different parts of the plant are eaten as a vegetable. The safest edible part of a legume is the seeds which are called pulses. Pulses include all beans, peas, and lentils. Examples of beans include navy, black, kidney, soy, green, pinto, fava and adzuki beans. Interestingly, the pod of the plant e.g., pea pods) where the seeds are stored can be eaten as well.

Why is it good for heart health?

The consumption of legumes is cardio-protective and reduces the risk of coronary heart disease (Marventano et al., 2017). 3-5 servings of legumes a week is associated with providing the most benefit to heart health (Marventano et al., 2017), (Safaeiyan et al, 2015). Research has found legume consumption to be effective in reducing LDL-cholesterol (the 'bad' cholesterol) in the blood due to its high soluble fibre content (Safaeiyan et al, 2015). When we ingest food, bile acids are released into the stomach and small intestine. Bile acids are produced in the liver from cholesterol and help us to digest food and nutrients. Soluble fibre interferes with bile being re-absorbed back into the liver. By blocking the re-absorption of bile, the liver draws cholesterol out of the blood, which in turn lowers blood cholesterol levels.

Top tips!

- Legumes are generally considered to be safe but need to be prepared and cooked properly. Some legumes, like soybeans and lentils, are known to have high levels of anti-nutrients called lectins (All recipes, 2022). These prevent nutrient absorption by the body and can be toxic if consumed in high amounts. Lectins are easy to get rid of; all you need to do is cook them. When heated past 212 degrees F (100 degrees C) for at least 30 minutes the lectins are destroyed (All, recipes, 2022). If you buy raw legumes, it is best to soak them for at least 5 hours in water to stay safe (All Recipes, 2022).

- Try to consume at least one portion (80g) of legumes every other day. Consuming legumes counts as a vegetable and therefore contributes towards your 5 a day.

- Legumes are great for soups, salads, pasta, and one-pot dishes.

- Legumes such as sugar snap peas make a great snack! Try to eat them in the most unprocessed form possible (apart from cooking for safety)

- Beans e.g., kidney and black-eyed beans can be cooked with rice.

- Black beans are a great addition to a burrito.

- Legumes are a good source of protein as well as a vegetable, so consider using them as a meat-free protein alternative in dishes. For example, lentils can be made to create shepherd's pie, cottage pie, burgers, casserole, and Bolognese.

- Make dhal by cooking lentils in Indian spices.

Recipe time!

Caribbean Pea Soup

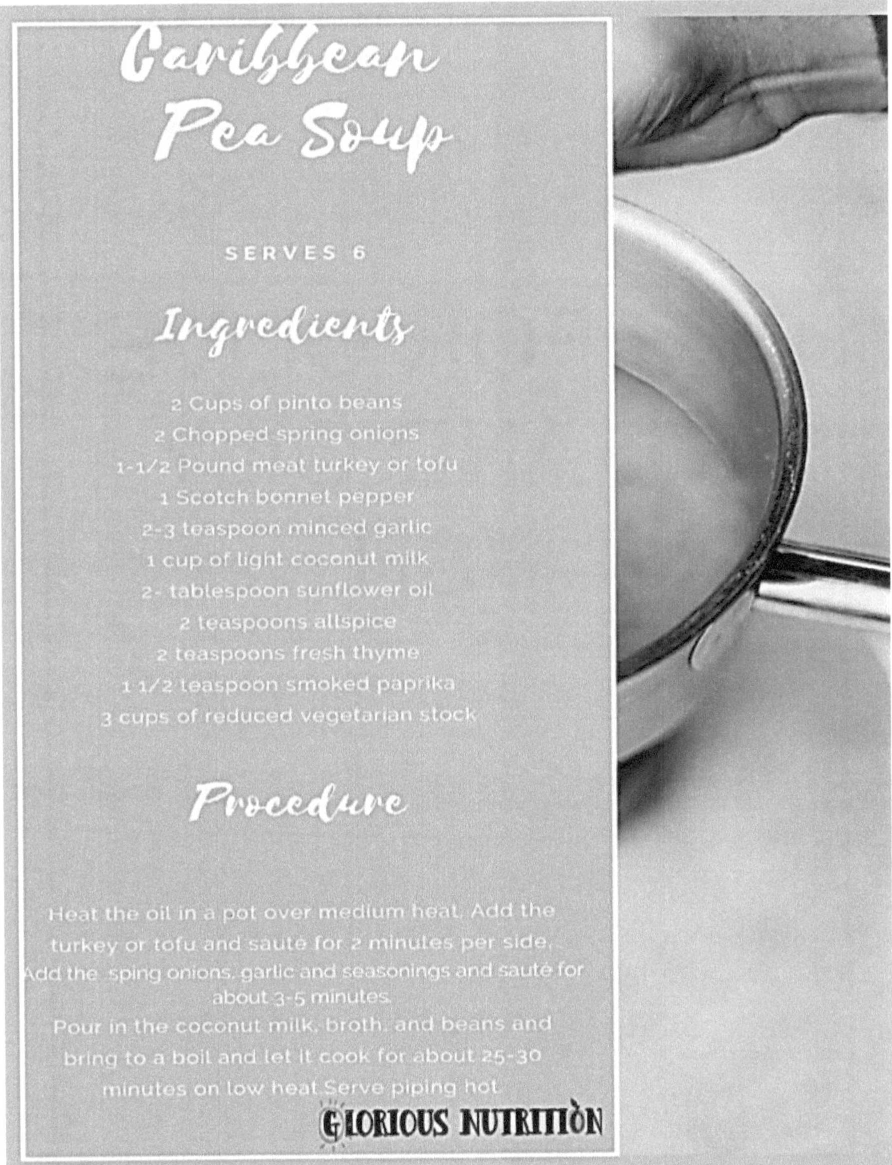

CHAPTER 12

O IS FOR OLIVE OIL AND OILY FISH

What is olive oil?

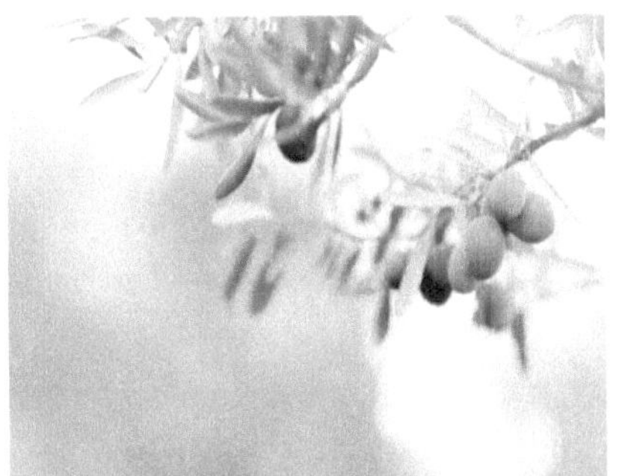

Olive oil is a liquid fat pressed from olives, the fruit of the olive tree. The olive tree originates from the Mediterranean basin.

Why is it good for heart health?

Olive oil consumption, especially the most unprocessed kind i.e., extra virgin olive oil (EVOO), has been shown to significantly reduce heart disease risk (Potì et al., 2019). Olive oil is a source of monounsaturated fatty acids, which have been found to increase the concentration of HDL (the 'good' cholesterol in the blood) and reduce the LDL: HDL ratio (Potì et al., 2019).

In addition, olive oil (apart from refined/processed olive oil) contains polyphenols with antioxidant properties (Potì et al., 2019). As mentioned previously, in heart health, polyphenols protect LDL molecules (the 'bad' cholesterol) from becoming unstable by interactions with polyphenols (unstable molecules in the environment) (Potì et al., 2019). When LDL molecules become unstable, by a process called oxidation, this cholesterol can become more reactive with the lining of blood vessels and promote atherosclerosis.

One study found that consuming more than 7 grams (>1/2 tablespoon) of olive oil per day was associated with a lower risk of heart disease mortality. Replacing margarine, butter, mayonnaise, and dairy fat with olive oil was associated with a lower risk of mortality (Guasch-Ferré et al., 2022).

Top tips!

- Consider using a tablespoon of extra virgin olive oil daily to soups, salads, stews, or on its own.

- You can even use virgin or extra virgin olive oil as an accompaniment with bread as a substitute for butter.

- For exploration, you can try spiced olive oil products such as olive oil with chilli flakes.

What is oily fish?

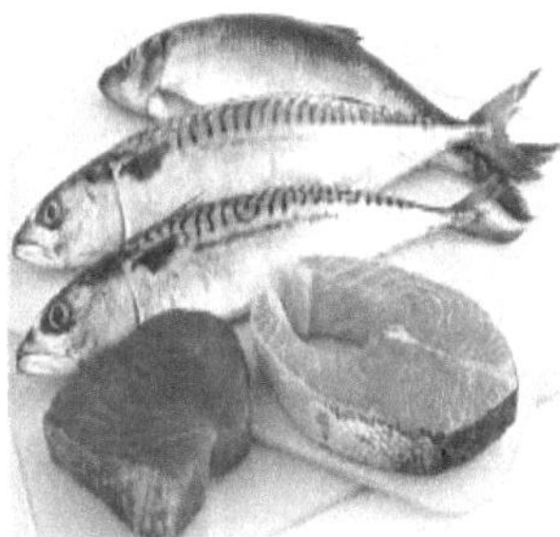

Oily fish are those that have oil distributed through their whole body, in contrast to white fish, whose main concentration of oils is in the liver. Examples of oily fish include salmon, mackerel, pilchards, sardines, herring, and trout.

Why is it good for heart health?

Oily fish are considered a major part of the Mediterranean diet which involves eating more bread, fruit, vegetables, fish, and less meat, and replacing butter with unsaturated fat spread. Research into this style of diet has been associated with a reduced risk of high blood pressure and raised blood cholesterol (Abdelhamid et al., 2020).

Oily fish is a good source of long-chain omega-3 fatty acids, which have been reported to improve heart health (Abdelhamid et al., 2020). Benefits include:

- Reductions in blood pressure

- Improvements in blood circulation

- A healthy blood lipid profile

Top tips!

- We should eat at least 1 portion (around 140g when cooked) of oily fish a week.

- If you are pregnant, planning to get pregnant, or breastfeeding, you should eat no more than two portions of oily fish per week. Avoid shark, marlin, and swordfish altogether. This is because oily fish contain more mercury than other types of fish.

- Oily fish goes well with peeled tomato plums. Stew the fish and add brown bread or rice as an accompaniment.

- Oily fish can be a great addition to sandwiches or wraps.

- You can eat oily fish as part of a sushi dish, but there are a few things to consider:

  - Keep rice to a minimum as sushi rice is often made 'sticky' with a combination of vinegar, sugar and salt which raise your salt intake for the day. Just one teaspoon of soy sauce contributes about 10-15% of your recommended daily salt intake.

  - Avoid any deep-fried dishes or mayonnaise-heavy dishes.

  - A study by the International Journal of Hygiene and Environmental Health found that blood levels were higher in mercury with weekly consumption of certain fish, including tuna steak and sushi. Therefore, mind your sushi portions and perhaps have it as a treat every so often instead of weekly.

o Pregnant women should avoid eating sushi due to the potential mercury levels and bacteria that may be present (as the fish is uncooked).

CHAPTER 13

P IS FOR PLUMS

What are plums?

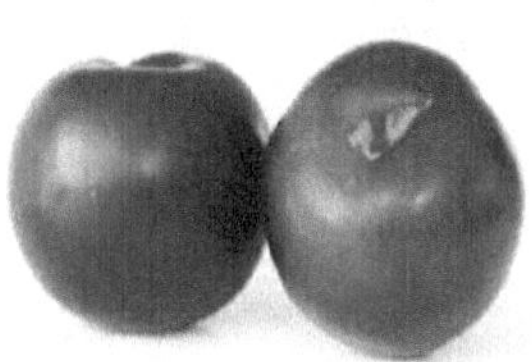

Plums are a type of stone fruit which is most commonly known for having dark purple-red skin, but plums can also be a green-yellow colour. The taste of plums ranges from sweet to sour. The best way to determine ripeness is to check the firmness rather than look for colour changes.

Why is it good for heart health?

Plums have a high phenolic content, mostly anthocyanins, which are known to be natural antioxidants (Igwe et al., 2016). Due to the high phenolic content, the consumption of plums has been reported to be associated with improvements in heart disease risk factors such as high blood pressure and blood cholesterol (Igwe et al., 2016).

Top tips!

- In line with general government guidance, try to eat at least five fruit and vegetables a day for health benefits.

- Plums make a pretty good snack! This will count towards your 5 a day.

- Once ripe, plums will keep at room temperature for around three to four days.

- Plums go well in overnight oats.

CHAPTER 14

R IS FOR RHUBARB

What is rhubarb?

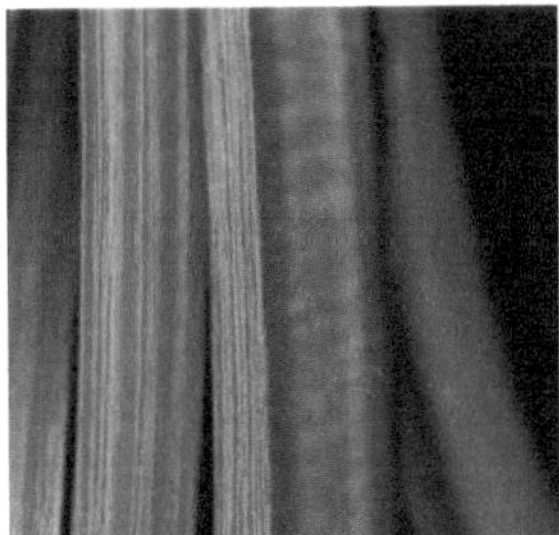

Rhubarb is a well-known traditional medicine. Rhubarb is a perennial with large green canopy leaves (which are inedible) and pink, red, or greenish fleshy, edible leaf stalks.

Why is it good for heart health?

Rhubarb is a rich source of fibre and antioxidants. Additionally, rhubarb contains anthraquinones and stilbenes which are compounds which have anti-inflammatory and blood-cholesterol-lowering effects (Liudvytska, 2022). Research has found that rhubarb stalk fibre has cholesterol-lowering effects and supports healthy artery function (Goel et al., 1997), (Liu et al., 2007).

Top tips!

- In line with general government guidance, try to eat at least five fruit and vegetables a day for health benefits.

- 5 canned chunks (in water) or 2 heaped tablespoons of rhubarb count towards your 5 a day.

- You can add rhubarb to plain yoghurt and low in sugar custard.

CHAPTER 15

S IS FOR SUNFLOWER SEEDS

What are sunflower seeds?

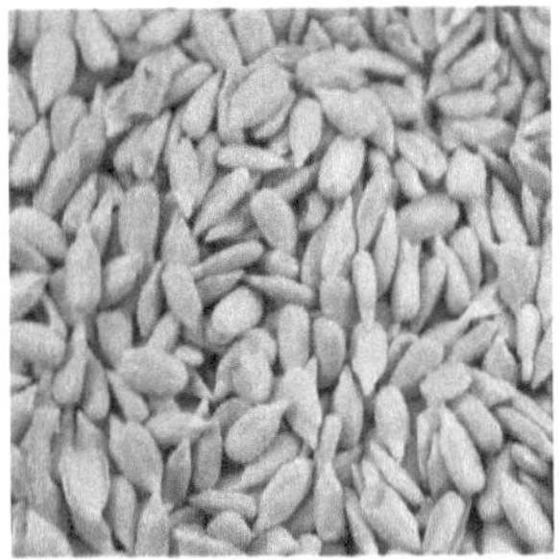 The sunflower seed is the seed/fruit of the sunflower plant (Helianthus annuus). Sunflower kernels are the edible part of the sunflower seed, which is revealed after the shell of the sunflower seed (called the hull) is removed.

Why is it good for heart health?

Nut and seed consumption is associated with a lower risk of heart disease in a dose-dependent manner i.e., the more you eat, the lower your heart disease risk (Arnesan et al., 2023). Sunflower seeds in particular are a good source of magnesium, fibre and heart-friendly fats including polyunsaturated fat and monounsaturated fat. Studies have shown that sunflower seeds are cardio-protective (Bester et al., 2010) (Kaur et al. 2021). For example, a study by Kaur et al. (2021) found that individuals who were provided with bread fortified with sunflower seed flour experienced weight loss and had improvements in their blood cholesterol profiles.

Top tips!

- You can sprinkle sunflower seeds over meals such as porridge, soup, salads, and stir-fries.

- You can eat a handful of sunflower seeds as a snack. Aim for around 2 tablespoons a day.

- You can add sunflower seeds to low in sugar energy balls.

CHAPTER 16

T IS FOR TUMERIC

What is turmeric?

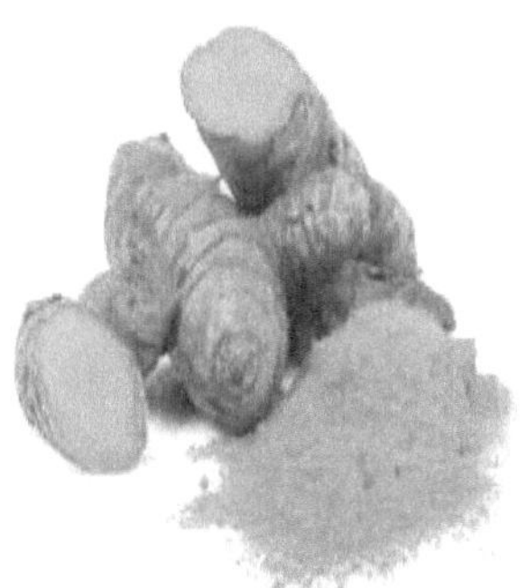

Turmeric is a herb that comes from the flowering turmeric plant. It has a warm, bitter taste and is often used in Asian cuisine. Turmeric is used as a spice & is a major component of a curry mix. The spice has a very vibrant colour, and it is often used as a colouring agent. The turmeric plant is native to the Indian subcontinent and Southeast Asia.

Why is it good for heart health?

Turmeric contains a yellow-coloured chemical called curcumin. This compound has been reported to be cardio-protective due to its lipid-lowering properties (Qin et al. 2017). A study assessed the efficacy and safety of turmeric and curcumin (extracted from turmeric) in lowering blood lipids in patients at risk of heart disease and found that both were effective at reducing blood cholesterol levels (Qin et al. 2017) (Hadi et al., 1019).

Top tips!

- If you would like to add turmeric to your diet, consume the spice with meals rather than on its own.

- You can add to curries, soups, rice dishes, salads, smoothies, hummus, roasted vegetables etc.

- Golden milk/turmeric latte- try turmeric and other spices heated with warm milk. You can make this and see how it tastes.

- For a serving recommendation and to avoid side effects, go for no more than 1 tablespoon a day.

CHAPTER 17

W IS FOR WALNUTS AND WHOLEGRAINS

What is a walnut?

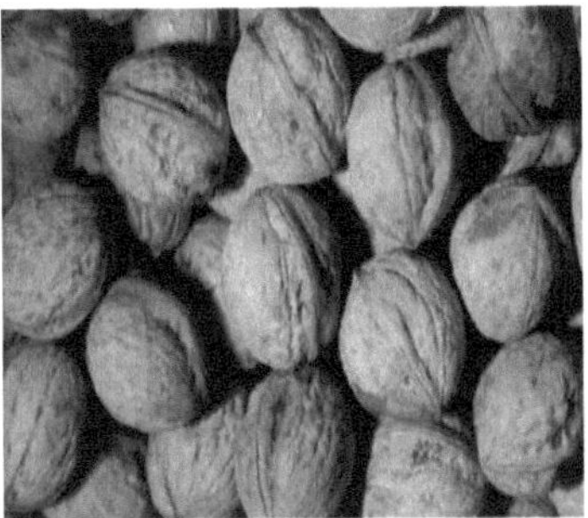

A walnut is a type of tree nut which has a globe-like shape and a hard shell. Walnuts are native to West Asia but are now produced in many countries including Turkey, the UK and the United States.

Why is it good for heart health?

There is strong evidence that nut consumption is protective against cardiovascular disease (Bonilla et al., 2018). Nuts are full of many nutrients and compounds that are beneficial to heart health (Bonilla et al., 2018). Walnuts have been identified as a nut that is particularly cardio-protective because they help to maintain healthy cholesterol levels and therefore keep the arteries healthy (Eslami et al., 2019). This is because walnuts are a rich source of alpha-linolenic acid (ALA) which as mentioned previously, is an essential omega-3 fatty acid. In studies, the consumption of walnuts has been found to reduce LDL cholesterol, the 'bad' cholesterol and reduce inflammation (Eslami et al., 2019). This is important because inflammation is a factor involved in the development of plaque build-up in the blood vessels i.e., atherosclerosis (Rock et al., 2017).

Top tips!

As mentioned in Chapter 3, there have been concerns about weight gain from eating nuts and seeds. However, there is no strong evidence that nuts eaten whole stimulate weight gain (Hollingworth et al., 2009). If you are concerned about weight gain, avoid nut butter and nuts coated in sugar, chocolate, salt, or honey-roasted varieties.

- A handful of whole nuts (about 30g) is a great filling snack. To add flavour, use spices and herbs (more details are available in Chapter 3 in the top tips section).

- Try adding a few walnuts to salads or soups.

- Sprinkle a few walnuts onto cereal or yoghurt.

What are wholegrains?

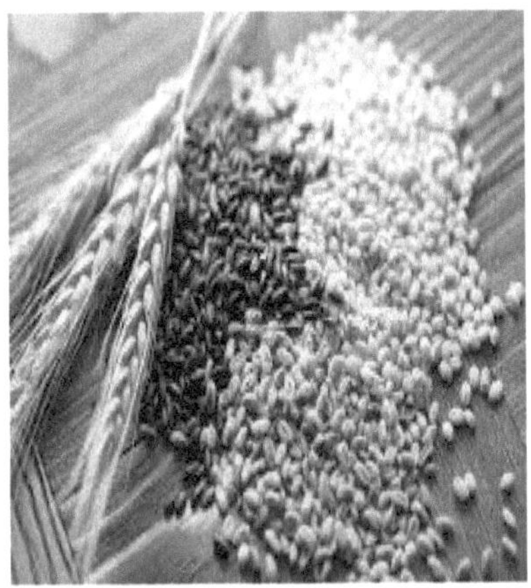

Grains are the seeds of grass-like plants called cereals. A huge variety of cereal crops are grown for food throughout the world including wheat, rye, barley, oats, and rice. A grain is considered to be a whole grain as long as all three original parts of a grain i.e., the bran, germ, and endosperm are still present.

Why is it good heart health?

There is evidence that wholegrain intake is associated with a reduced risk of coronary heart disease and cardiovascular disease. Whole grains are high in soluble fibre (oats, barley) which has been found to improve blood cholesterol, low-density lipoprotein cholesterol (LDL), blood pressure and insulin sensitivity (Dagfinn et al., 2016). In addition, wholegrains are also high in insoluble fibre which has been reported to have the ability to also reduce blood pressure (Dagfinn et al., 2016).

Top tips!

- Swap white bread/tortilla wraps for wholegrain bread for toast and sandwiches.

- Choose wholegrain varieties of rice, pasta, noodles, cous cous, buckwheat, and quinoa.

- Look out for the 100% wholegrain stamp on products.

CHAPTER 18

DECISION TIME

So, we have come to the end of discussing foods that are argued by research to be cardio-protective in nature and therefore, likely to be beneficial to heart health. Hope you enjoyed it! After reviewing the reported cardio-protective foods against the criteria, 7 foods made the food alphabet for heart health checklist.

The criteria to make the checklist were deliberately strict and food items had to meet at least three of the following standards:

- The food item had to be well-researched.
- The food item had to be a whole food i.e., unprocessed or unrefined with the exception of a food item being drained or cooked for safety purposes.
- The evidence on the heart health benefits of the food item had to be from the highest forms of evidence (level 1). These currently are systematic reviews and meta-analyses. For more information about these types of research, please have a look at this website:

- The findings around the heart health benefits of the food items had to be consistent.

Please see Figure 1 below which provides a summary of the food alphabet in the form of a checklist.

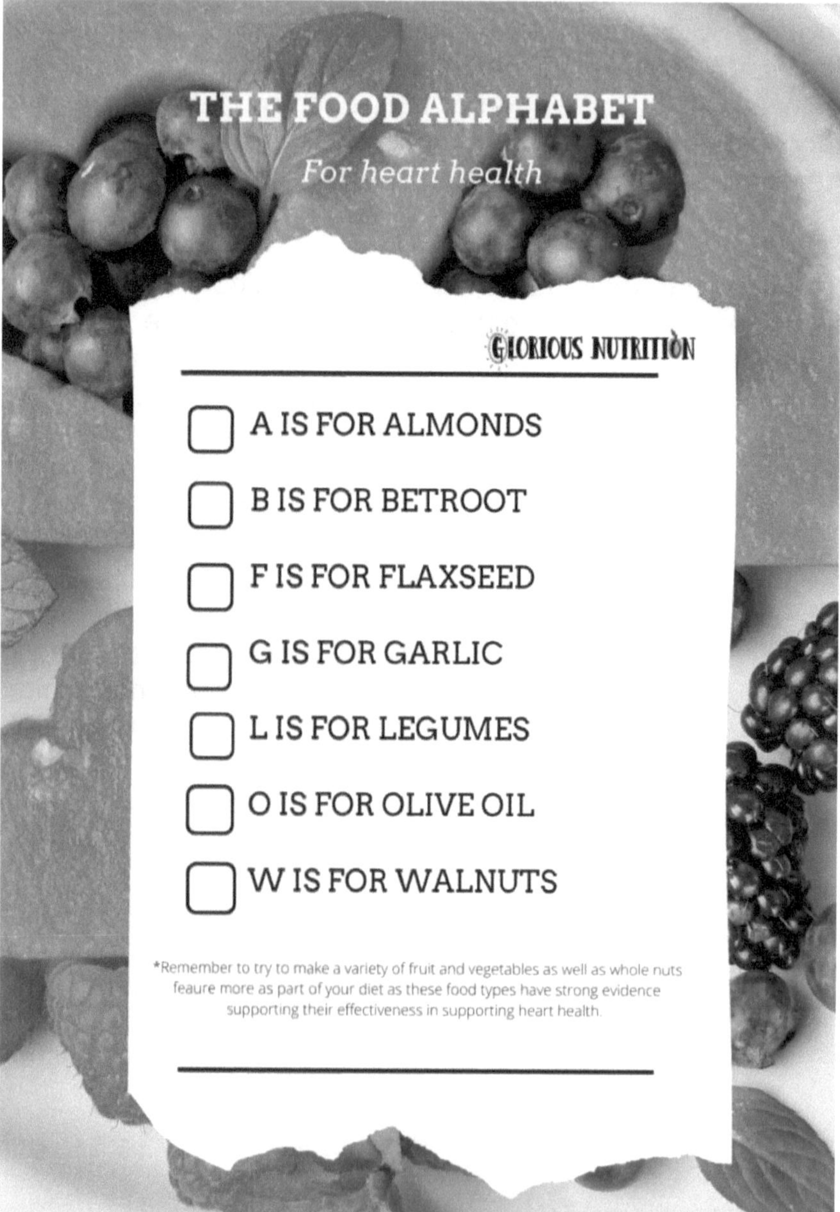

With this food alphabet checklist, you can hopefully look forward to the main benefits:

- A reduction in heart disease risk
- A healthy reduction in blood pressure
- Healthier blood cholesterol levels
- Protection from artery blood vessel damage
- Reduced inflammation

Please see a list of food items that didn't meet the eligibility criteria for the food alphabet for heart health checklist, **but do appear to be beneficial** to heart health and can be added to your diet:
- Berries
- Cinnamon
- Dairy
- Dark chocolate
- Eggplant
- Kale
- Oily fish
- Plums
- Rhubarb
- Sunflower
- Turmeric
- Wholegrains

CHAPTER 19

OTHER LIFESTYLE FACTORS

Foods to avoid

Foods high in sugar, animal fat, hydrogenated fat (i.e., Trans-Fats) and/or salt should be limited in the diet. Foods that tend to have a combination of these nutrients are processed and ultra-processed 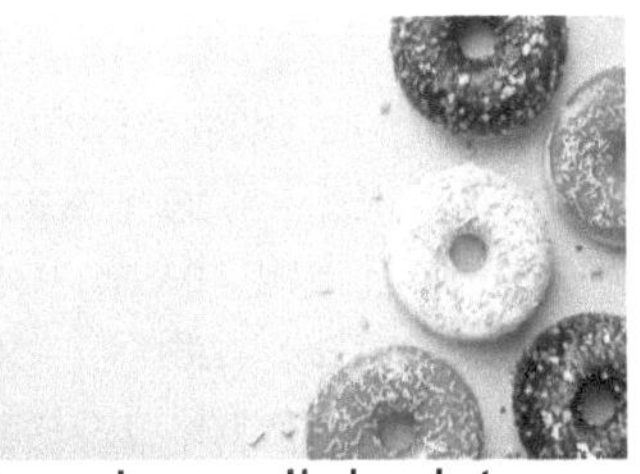 foods. Consumption of such foods has been linked to an increased risk of heart disease (Micha et al., 2010). Examples include processed meats (bacon, deli meats, hot dogs etc.), highly refined and processed grains and carbohydrates (white bread, white rice, and low-fibre breakfast cereals) & soft drinks and other sugary drinks. It is suggested that they may affect cardiometabolic health by negatively influencing digestion, appetite regulation, bacteria in the gut and the body's response to sugar (Juul et al., 2021). In addition, there is overwhelming evidence that dietary salt is a major cause of raised blood pressure (He et al., 2007).

Mental health and wellness

It is important to look after your mental health & well-being, especially due to stress management, because poor mental health can be significantly harmful to heart health (Esler, 2017). There is increasing evidence that 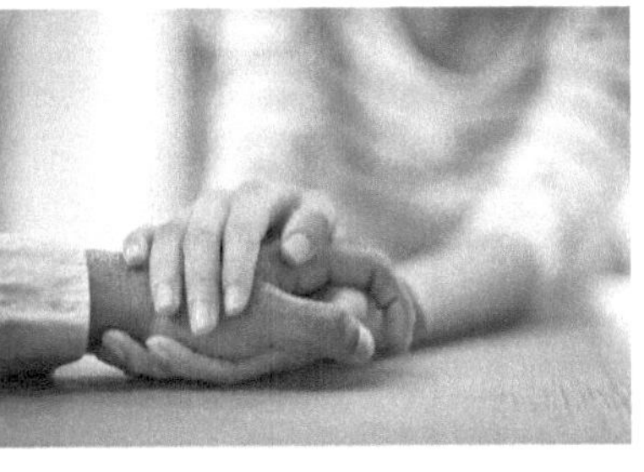 psychological health may be causally linked to biological processes and behaviours that contribute to and cause heart disease (Levine et al, 2021). For instance, emotional stress (acute or chronic) has been found to increase the risk of heart disease and acute coronary heart disease events (Wirtz et al., 2017).

Quitting smoking/tobacco use

Smoking is one of the top causes of heart disease and has been found to damage arteries and increase blood pressure. Research has even established that cigarette smoking can increase the risk of death from CVD by up to three times (National Heart, Lung and Blood, Institute, 2022). If you already have coronary heart disease, quitting smoking greatly lowers your risk of having more heart attacks or dying from that heart disease (by up to 50% or more) (Jha et.al, 2013). Second-hand smoke is also harmful, and evidence has shown that exposure to second-hand smoke increases the risk of heart disease by 23% (Lv et al., 2015) and specifically increases ischemic and coronary heart disease risk by 25–30% (Dunbar et al., 2013).

Limiting alcohol

What is known for certain, is that heavy consumption has been associated with unfavourable cardiovascular outcomes including increased mortality (Goel., et al 2018) (Biddinger et al., 2022). There's a popular belief that alcohol, especially red wine, is good for the heart, but the evidence to support this is not fully clear. Therefore, it is best to reduce your alcohol consumption and at the very least keep within the guidelines of no more than 14 units of alcohol each week and several alcohol-free days (NHS, 2021). One unit is equivalent to 8 grams/10 ml of pure alcohol (NHS, 2021).

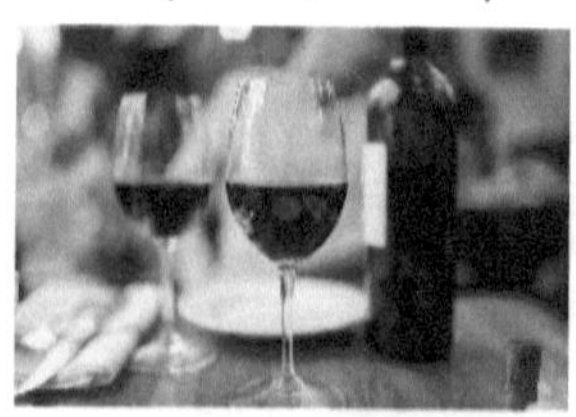

Gum inflammation

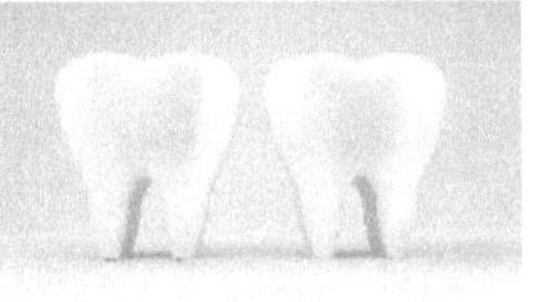

It is important to maintain good oral hygiene to reduce your risk of gum inflammation. Good oral health practices include brushing your teeth twice a day with fluoride toothpaste and spitting, not rinsing (NHS, 2022). In addition, regularly flossing and using interdental brushes to clean debris in between teeth (NHS, 2022). Regular check-ups with the dentist are crucial too (NHS, 2022). A build of plaque along the gum line can lead to inflammation of the gums due to the many types of harmful bacteria found in plaque (Vera-Pineda et al. 2018). Periodontal inflammation is associated with an increased risk of heart disease (especially coronary heart disease) (Gao et al., 2021) (Priyamvara et al., 2020). The mechanism is still under investigation, but it is believed that periodontal inflammation drives atherosclerosis by causing bacterial growth over atherosclerotic plaques (Priyamvara et al., 2020).

Sleep Quality

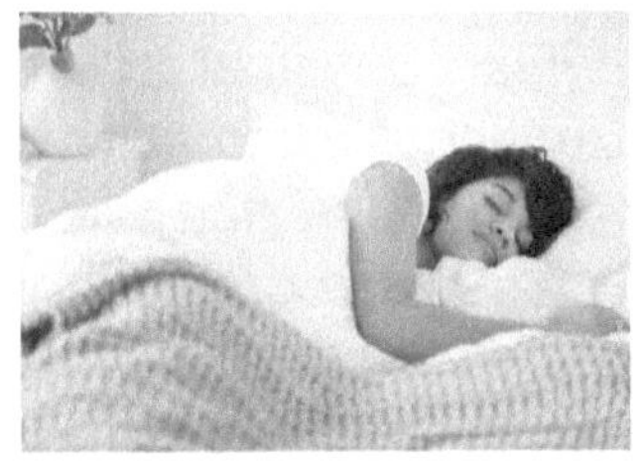

Getting enough sleep is paramount to leading a healthy and productive lifestyle and it is recommended that on average adults need between 7-9 hours of sleep a night (NHS, 2021). Research has found that sleep disorders, especially chronic shortened sleep, are a risk factor for heart disease and may contribute towards atherosclerotic burden and put an individual more at risk of developing other risk factors such as obesity and hypertension (Sadabadi et al., 2023), (Laksono et al., 2022). If you are struggling with your sleep, try to make your time before bed & sleep environment as relaxing as possible. Please speak to your doctor for further support.

Physical activity

Being physically active is beneficial to our health and wellness in many ways. It is recommended that adults should do at least 150–300 minutes of moderate-intensity aerobic physical activity; or at least 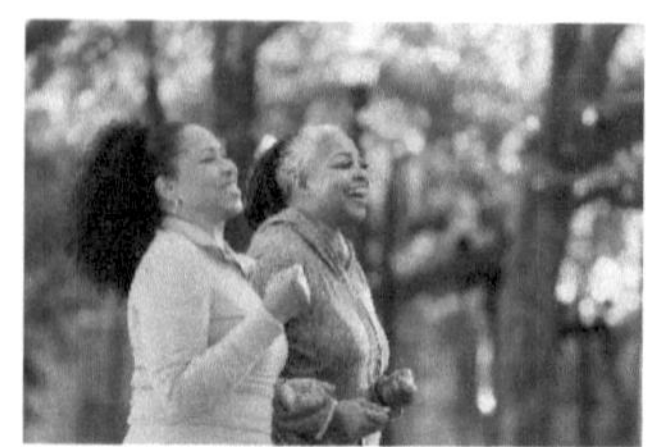 75–150 minutes of vigorous-intensity aerobic physical activity; or an equivalent combination of moderate- and vigorous-intensity activity throughout the week (World Health Organization, 2022). Muscle-strengthening activities at a moderate or greater intensity that involve all major muscle groups on 2 or more days a week are also recommended. Research has found that increases in regular physical activity are linked to reduced cardiovascular risk and mortality. Additionally, meeting the recommendations for muscle-strengthening exercises, if you were previously inactive, is associated with improved cardiovascular outcomes (Lanier et al., 2016) (Pinckard et al., 2019). Physical activity reduces cardiometabolic risk factors (i.e., high blood pressure, high blood cholesterol, obesity, uncontrolled blood glucose etc.). Some mechanisms in which physical activity supports health is by improving cell function, restoration and improvement of blood vessels, and the release of myokines (small proteins released because of muscular contractions) from skeletal muscle that preserves cardiovascular function (Pinckard et al., 2019).

A lot of people anecdotally report that they struggle to exercise due to busy schedules and costs. A great affordable form of exercise to try out is completing regular brisk walks. Walking is simple and there are plenty of apps to help you keep on track of your steps. Also, just by being more aware of opportunities to be active, you can squeeze exercise in. For instance, taking the stairs instead of the lift, walking part way to work and completing seat exercises while watching TV. Speak to an exercise professional for tailored advice.

CHAPTER 20

CLOSING REMARKS

The power of nutrition can truly be powerful and glorious, and this is especially true for heart health. Many people have seen dramatic changes in their health just by diet alone. With this being said, it is important that you stay safe and therefore, I would encourage you to speak to a health professional before making any drastic changes to heart health medication and any other significant changes to your heart disease treatment.

I haven't focused heavily on what you should avoid eating in this book, but it is very much in line with the general healthy eating guidance. For heart health and overall health, it is important that your diet is low in refined grains, trans-fats, and added sugars including sugar-sweetened beverages and red and processed meats. In contrast, please try to follow a diet that focuses on the right balance of fruits and vegetables, legumes, nuts, fish (especially oily fish), poultry, wholegrains, moderate dairy, and heart-healthy vegetable oils such as olive oil. Please omit the relevant food items just mentioned if you are vegan or vegetarian with suitable alternatives.

Remember, along with eating well for heart health, you should practice a healthy lifestyle which includes the following:

- Regular physical activity
- Looking after your mental health (especially regarding effective stress management)
- Quitting smoking/tobacco use
- Limiting alcohol
- Making sleep a priority

Why not take the challenge of repeating the healthy eating quiz after 6 weeks and see if you can improve your score? You will find in the next Chapter (Chapter 21,) other useful tools and resources to help you on your heart health journey.

Thank you for taking the time to read this book and now after reading it, I hope you feel more knowledgeable about what to eat for heart health. For useful nutritional resources and support, please visit the Glorious Nutrition (GN) website (see link below). Also, please feel free to stay connected by following GN on social media.

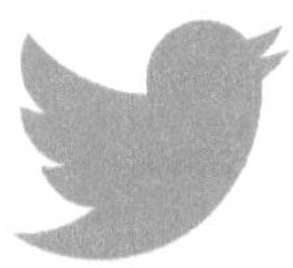 @gloriousnutri1

 @FeelGloriousNutritionConsulting

 @gloriousnutrition5

 https://gloriousnutr.wordpress.com/

CHAPTER 21

TOOLS AND RESOURCES

Cardioprotective 5-day meal plan

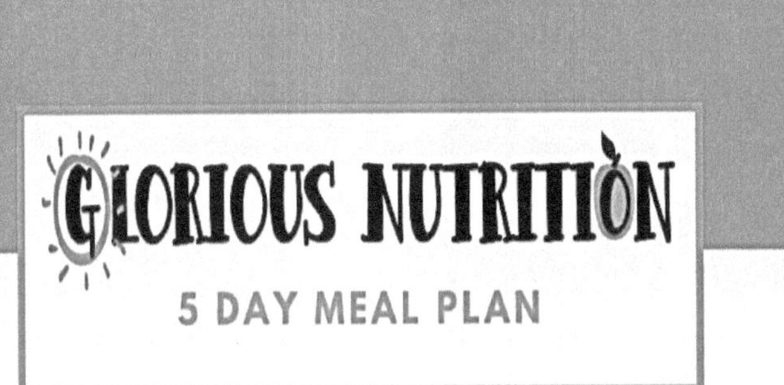

MONDAY

Beans on brown toast, Wholemeal turkey Wrap
1 apple, Spicy Chicken and Pasta, Side salad and 2 Tbsp olive oil

TUESDAY

No added sugar walnut & almond museli with semi-skimmed milk, Betroot salad with feta cheese, Black bean soup

WEDNESDAY

Porridge with berries, Veggie Bean Burger and wholemeal Bun, Seared salmon with turmeric spiced baby potatoes & green beans

THURSDAY

Roasted plum breakfast parfait, Pesto pasta, Chickpea & sweet potato curry with tumeric brown rice

FRIDAY

Yoghurt with berry compote, walnut salad, chilli con carne with extra kidney beans and garlic rice

SATURDAY

Loaded Vegetable Omelet, Garlic toast, fruit salad, Chicken with an extra virgin olive oil dressing with carrots

Setting SMART goals

How do you plan to incorporate the food alphabet checklist into your diet? One way to ensure that what you have learnt has to be put into action is to set SMART goals (Doran, 1981).

SMART stands for **S**pecific, Measurable, **A**chievable, **R**ealistic, and **T**imely.

Example: I will have a <u>handful</u> of <u>almonds</u> <u>once a day for the next 6 months and review.</u>

1.

2.

3.

4.

5.

Progress after 1 month, 3 months, 6 months, a year……

1.

2.

3.

4.

92

5.

Blood Pressure Log

As a general guide:
Ideal blood pressure is considered to be between 90/60mmHg and 120/80mmH. If you are anxious or stressed, this can affect the reading. You can check your blood pressure at any time and if you have been diagnosed with or are at risk of developing high blood pressure, you may need more frequent checks of your blood pressure.

Date	Time	Systolic	Diastolic	Notes

Date	Time	Systolic	Diastolic	Notes

Other support and resources

Fitness

Portion size guidance

Alcohol management

Quitting smoking/tobacco usage

Mental wellness & sleep

CHAPTER 22

REFERENCES AND INDEX

References

1. Abdelhamid AS, Brown TJ, Brainard JS, Biswas P, Thorpe GC, Moore HJ, Deane KHO, Summerbell CD, Worthington HV, Song F, Hooper L. Omega-3 fatty acids for the primary and secondary prevention of cardiovascular disease. Cochrane Database of Systematic Reviews 2020, Issue 3. Art. No.: CD003177. DOI: 10.1002/14651858.CD003177.pub5.

2. All, recipes. (2022) The Dangers of uncooked beans and Lentils. Does Eating Raw or Undercooked Beans and Lentils Cause Food Poisoning? (allrecipes.com) Accessed 15.05.23.

3. Anand SS, Hawkes C, de Souza RJ, et al. Food Consumption and its Impact on Cardiovascular Disease: Importance of Solutions Focused on the Globalized Food System: A Report From the Workshop Convened by the World Heart Federation. *J Am Coll Cardiol*. 2015;66(14):1590-1614. doi:10.1016/j.jacc.2015.07.050

4. Arnesen EK, Thorisdottir B, Bärebring L, Söderlund F, Nwaru BI, Spielau U, Dierkes J, Ramel A, Lamberg-Allardt C, Åkesson A. Nuts and seeds consumption and risk of cardiovascular disease, type 2 diabetes and their risk factors: a systematic review and meta-analysis. Food Nutr Res. 2023 Feb 14;67. doi: 10.29219/fnr.v67.8961. PMID: 36816545; PMCID: PMC9930735.

5. Aune Dagfinn, Keum NaNa, Giovannucci Edward, Fadnes Lars T, Boffetta Paolo, Greenwood Darren C et al. Whole grain consumption and risk of cardiovascular disease, cancer, and all-cause and cause-specific mortality: a systematic review and dose-response meta-analysis of prospective studies BMJ 2016; 353:i2716

6. Basu A, Rhone M, Lyons TJ. Berries: emerging impact on cardiovascular health. Nutr Rev. 2010;68(3):168-177. doi:10.1111/j.1753-4887.2010.00273.x

7. Bester D, Esterhuyse AJ, Truter EJ, van Rooyen J. Cardiovascular effects of edible oils: a comparison between four popular edible oils. Nutr Res Rev. 2010 Dec;23(2):334-48. doi 10.1017/S0954422410000223. Epub 2010 Sep 20. PMID: 20849681.

8. Better Health Channel. (2022). Cholesterol. Cholesterol - Better Health Channel Accessed 14.05.2023.

9. Biddinger KJ, Emdin CA, Haas ME, et al. Association of Habitual Alcohol Intake With Risk of Cardiovascular Disease. JAMA Netw Open. 2022;5(3):e223849. doi:10.1001/jamanetworkopen.2022.3849

10. Bonilla Ocampo DA, Paipilla AF, Marín E, Vargas-Molina S, Petro JL, Pérez-Idárraga A. Dietary Nitrate from Beetroot Juice for Hypertension: A Systematic

Review. Biomolecules. 2018;8(4):134. Published 2018 Nov 2. doi:10.3390/biom8040134

11. Carrizales-Sepúlveda EF, Ordaz-Farías A, Vera-Pineda R, Flores-Ramírez R. Periodontal Disease, Systemic Inflammation and the Risk of Cardiovascular Disease. Heart Lung Circ. 2018 Nov;27(11):1327-1334. doi 10.1016/j.hlc.2018.05.102. Epub 2018 Jun 2. PMID: 29903685.

12. Centers for Disease and Control and Prevention (CDC). CDC Prevention Programmes 2018. Available from:https://www.heart.org/en/get-involved/advocate/federal-priorities/cdc-prevention-programs Accessed: 05.05.20

13. Charis M.G. 2021. Nutraceutical and Functional Food Components. *Effects of Innovative Processing Techniques* https://doi.org/10.1016/C2020-0-02099-2

14. Das S, Raychaudhuri U, Falchi M, Bertelli A, Braga PC, Das DK. Cardioprotective properties of raw and cooked eggplant (Solanum melongena L). Food Funct. 2011 Jul;2(7):395-9. doi: 10.1039/c1fo10048c. Epub 2011 Jun 10. PMID: 21894326.

15. de Souza RGM, Schincaglia RM, Pimentel GD, Mota JF. Nuts and Human Health Outcomes: A Systematic Review. Nutrients. 2017;9(12):1311. Published 2017 Dec 2. doi:10.3390/nu9121311

16. Diabetes UK. Complications of diabetes. Complications of diabetes | Guide to diabetes | Diabetes UK Accessed 14.05.2023.

17. Dm coffee blog (2022) Does dark chocolate contain flavonoids? Does dark chocolate contain flavonoids? – Dmcoffee.blog Accessed 21.05.23

18. *Doran, G. T. (1981). "There's a S.M.A.R.T. Way to Write Management's Goals and Objectives", Management Review, Vol. 70, Issue 11, pp. 35-36.*

19. Dunbar A, Gotsis W, Frishman W. Second-hand tobacco smoke and cardiovascular disease risk: an epidemiological review. Cardiology in review. 2013; 21(2):94–100.

20. EFSA Panel on Food Contact Materials, Enzymes, Flavourings and Processing Aids, 2004. Opinion of the Scientific Panel on food additives, flavourings, processing aids and materials in contact with food (AFC) related to Coumarin. *EFSA Journal* 2004; 2(12):104, 36 pp. doi:10.2903/j.efsa.2004.104.

21. Eslami O, Shidfar F, Dehnad A. Inverse association of long-term nut consumption with weight gain and risk of overweight/obesity: a systematic review. *Nutr Res.* 2019;68:1-8. doi:10.1016/j.nutres.2019.04.001

22. Esler M. Mental stress and human cardiovascular disease. Neurosci Biobehav Rev. 2017 Mar;74(Pt

B):269-276. doi: 10.1016/j.neubiorev.2016.10.011. Epub 2016 Oct 14. PMID: 27751732.

23. Faezeh Askari, Bahram Rashidkhani, Azita Hekmatdoost. (2014) Cinnamon may have therapeutic benefits on lipid profile, liver enzymes, insulin resistance, and high-sensitivity C-reactive protein in nonalcoholic fatty liver disease patients. Nutrition Research, Volume 34, Issue 2. https://doi.org/10.1016/j.nutres.2013.11.005.

24. Faridi Z, Njike VY, Dutta S, Ali A, Katz DL. Acute dark chocolate and cocoa ingestion and endothelial function: a randomized controlled crossover trial. Am J Clin Nutr. 2008 Jul;88(1):58-63. doi: 10.1093/ajcn/88.1.58. PMID: 18614724.

25. Feingold KR, Grunfeld C. Introduction to Lipids and Lipoproteins. [Updated 2018 Feb 2]. In: Feingold KR, Anawalt B, Boyce A, et al., editors. Endotext [Internet]. South Dartmouth (MA): MDText.com, Inc.; 2000-. Available from: https://www.ncbi.nlm.nih.gov/books/NBK305896/ Accessed 11.06.20.

26. Fisher ND, Hughes M, Gerhard-Herman M, Hollenberg NK. Flavanol-rich cocoa induces nitric-oxide-dependent vasodilation in healthy humans. J Hypertens. 2003 Dec;21(12):2281-6. doi: 10.1097/00004872-200312000-00016. PMID: 14654748.

27. Gao S, Tian J, Li Y, Liu T, Li R, Yang L, Xing Z. Periodontitis and Number of Teeth in the Risk of Coronary Heart Disease: An Updated Meta-Analysis. Med Sci Monit. 2021 Aug 23;27:e930112. doi: 10.12659/MSM.930112. PMID: 34421117; PMCID: PMC8394608.

28. George ES, Marshall S, Mayr HL, et al. The effect of high-polyphenol extra virgin olive oil on cardiovascular risk factors: A systematic review and meta-analysis. Crit Rev Food Sci Nutr. 2019;59(17):2772-2795. doi:10.1080/10408398.2018.1470491.

29. Goel S, Sharma A, Garg A. Effect of Alcohol Consumption on Cardiovascular Health. Curr Cardiol Rep. 2018 Mar 8;20(4):19. doi 10.1007/s11886-018-0962-2. PMID: 29520541.

30. Goel V, Ooraikul B, Basu TK. Cholesterol-lowering effects of rhubarb stalk fiber in hypercholesterolemic men. J Am Coll Nutr. 1997 Dec;16(6):600-604. PMID: 9430089.

31. Guasch-Ferré M, Li Y, Willett W, et al. Consumption of Olive Oil and Risk of Total and Cause-Specific Mortality Among U.S. Adults. J Am Coll Cardiol. 2022 Jan, 79 (2) 101–112. https://doi.org/10.1016/j.jacc.2021.10.041

32. Guimarães P, Galvão A, Batista C, Azevedo G, Oliveira R, Lamounier R, et al. Eggplant (Solanum

melongena) infusion has a modest and transitory effect on hypercholesterolemic subjects. *Braz J Med Biol Res.* 2000;33:1027–1036.

33. Hadi A, Pourmasoumi M, Ghaedi E, Sahebkar A. The effect of Curcumin/Turmeric on blood pressure modulation: A systematic review and meta-analysis. Pharmacol Res. 2019 Dec;150:104505. doi: 10.1016/j.phrs.2019.104505. Epub 2019 Oct 21. PMID: 31647981.

34. He FJ, MacGregor GA. Salt, blood pressure and cardiovascular disease. Curr Opin Cardiol. 2007 Jul;22(4):298-305. doi 10.1097/HCO.0b013e32814f1d8c. PMID: 17556881.

35. Heiss C, Finis D, Kleinbongard P, Hoffmann A, Rassaf T, Kelm M, Sies H. Sustained increase in flow-mediated dilation after daily intake of high-flavanol cocoa drink over 1 week. J Cardiovasc Pharmacol. 2007 Feb;49(2):74-80. doi: 10.1097/FJC.0b013e31802d0001. PMID: 17312446.

36. Hollingworth S, Dalton M, Blundell JE, Finlayson G. Evaluation of the Influence of Raw Almonds on Appetite Control: Satiation, Satiety, Hedonics and Consumer Perceptions. *Nutrients.* 2019;11(9):2030. Published 2019 Aug 30. doi:10.3390/nu11092030

37. British Heart Foundation. Oily fish. https://www.bhf.org.uk/informationsupport/heart-matters-magazine/nutrition/oily-fish. Accessed 22.05.2023.

38. Igwe, Ezinne & Charlton, Karen. (2016). A Systematic Review on the Health Effects of Plums (Prunus domestica and Prunus salicina). Phytotherapy Research. 30. n/a-n/a. 10.1002/ptr.5581.

39. Jha P, Ramasundarahettige C, Landsman V, Rostron B, Thun M, Anderson RN, McAfee T, Peto R. 21st-century hazards of smoking and benefits of cessation in the United States. New England Journal of Medicine. 2013 Jan 24;368(4):341-50

40. Juul F, Vaidean G, Parekh N. Ultra-processed Foods and Cardiovascular Diseases: Potential Mechanisms of Action. Adv Nutr. 2021 Oct 1;12(5):1673-1680. doi: 10.1093/advances/nmab049. PMID: 33942057; PMCID: PMC8483964.

41. Kaur G, Kaur N, Kaur A. Lipid profile of hyperlipidemic males after supplementation of multigrain bread containing sunflower (*Helianthus annuus*) seed flour. J Food Sci Technol. 2021 Jul;58(7):2617-2629. doi: 10.1007/s13197-020-04768-w. Epub 2020 Sep 26. PMID: 34194097; PMCID: PMC8196128.

42. Khan A, Safdar M, Ali Khan MM, Khattak KN, Anderson RA. Cinnamon improves glucose and lipids of people with type 2 diabetes. Diabetes Care. 2003 Dec;26(12):3215-8. doi: 10.2337/diacare.26.12.3215. PMID: 14633804.

43. Kim SY, Yoon S, Kwon SM, Park KS, Lee-Kim YC. Kale juice improves coronary artery disease risk factors in hypercholesterolemic men. Biomed Environ Sci. 2008 Apr;21(2):91-7. doi: 10.1016/S0895-3988(08)60012-4. PMID: 18548846.

44. Laksono S, Yanni M, Iqbal M, Prawara AS. Abnormal Sleep Duration as Predictor for Cardiovascular Diseases: A Systematic Review of Prospective Studies. Sleep Disord. 2022 Feb 7;2022:9969107. doi: 10.1155/2022/9969107. PMID: 35178257; PMCID: PMC8844105.

45. Lanier JB, Bury DC, Richardson SW. Diet and Physical Activity for Cardiovascular Disease Prevention. Am Fam Physician. 2016 Jun 1;93(11):919-24. PMID: 27281836.

46. Lee-Bravatti MA, Wang J, Avendano EE, King L, Johnson EJ, Raman G. Almond Consumption and Risk Factors for Cardiovascular Disease: A Systematic Review and Meta-analysis of Randomized Controlled Trials. Adv Nutr. 2019;10(6):1076-1088. doi:10.1093/advances/nmz043.

47. Levine GN, Cohen BE, Commodore-Mensah Y, Fleury J, Huffman JC, Khalid U, Labarthe DR, Lavretsky H, Michos ED, Spatz ES, Kubzansky LD. Psychological Health, Well-Being, and the Mind-Heart-Body Connection: A Scientific Statement From the American Heart Association. Circulation. 2021 Mar 9;143(10):e763-e783. doi:

10.1161/CIR.0000000000000947. Epub 2021 Jan 25. PMID: 33486973.

48. Liu YF, Yu HM, Zhang C, Yan FF, Liu Y, Zhang Y, Zhang M, Zhao YX. Treatment with rhubarb improves brachial artery endothelial function in patients with atherosclerosis: a randomized, double-blind, placebo-controlled clinical trial. Am J Chin Med. 2007;35(4):583-95. doi: 10.1142/S0192415X07005089. PMID: 17708625.

49. Liudvytska O, Kolodziejczyk-Czepas J. A Review on Rhubarb-Derived Substances as Modulators of Cardiovascular Risk Factors-A Special Emphasis on Anti-Obesity Action. Nutrients. 2022 May 13;14(10):2053. doi: 10.3390/nu14102053. PMID: 35631194; PMCID: PMC9144273.

50. Luís Â , Domingues F , Pereira L . Association between berries intake and cardiovascular diseases risk factors: a systematic review with meta-analysis and trial sequential analysis of randomized controlled trials. Food Funct. 2018;9(2):740-757. doi:10.1039/c7fo01551h.

51. Lv X, Sun J, Bi Y, Xu M, Lu J, Zhao L, Xu Y. Risk of all-cause mortality and cardiovascular disease associated with secondhand smoke exposure: a systematic review and meta-analysis. International journal of cardiology. 2015 Nov 15;199:106-15.

52. Marventano S, Izquierdo Pulido M, Sánchez-González C, et al. Legume consumption and CVD risk: a systematic review and meta-analysis. *Public Health Nutr.* 2017;20(2):245-254. doi:10.1017/S1368980016002299.

53. Micha R, Wallace SK, Mozaffarian D. Red and processed meat consumption and risk of incident coronary heart disease, stroke, and diabetes mellitus: a systematic review and meta-analysis. Circulation. 2010 Jun 1;121(21):2271-83. doi: 10.1161/CIRCULATIONAHA.109.924977. Epub 2010 May 17. PMID: 20479151; PMCID: PMC2885952.

54. Mollazadeh H, Hosseinzadeh H. Cinnamon effects on metabolic syndrome: a review based on its mechanisms. Iran J Basic Med Sci. 2016 Dec;19(12):1258-1270. doi: 10.22038/ijbms.2016.7906. PMID: 28096957; PMCID: PMC5220230.

55. Mozaffarian D and Wu JHY. Flavonoids, dairy foods, and cardiovascular and metabolic health: A review of emerging biologic pathways. Circ Res 2018;122:369-384.

56. National Heart, Lung and Blood, Institute. (2022). Benefits of Quitting Smoking. Smoking and Your Heart - Benefits of Quitting Smoking | NHLBI, NIH Accessed 15.05.23.

57. NCD Alliance, Cardiovascular Disease Cardiovascular Diseases | NCD Alliance. Accessed 09.05.23.

58. NHS. (2021) Alcohol units. Alcohol units - NHS (www.nhs.uk) Accessed 16.05.23.

59. NHS. (2021). Insomnia. Insomnia - NHS (www.nhs.uk) Accessed 17.05.23.

60. NHS. (2022) Preventing Gum Disease. Gum disease - NHS (www.nhs.uk). Accessed 17.05.23.

61. NHS. (2022). Metabolic Syndrome. Metabolic syndrome - NHS (www.nhs.uk) Accessed 14.05.2023.

62. NHS. (2023). High Blood Pressure (Hypertension). High blood pressure (hypertension) - NHS (www.nhs.uk) Accessed 14.05.2023.

63. Noia J.D. Defining powerhouse fruits and vegetables: A nutrient density approach. *Prev. Chronic Dis.* 2014;11:1–5.

64. Obermeyer, W. R., Musser, S. M., Betz, J. M., Casey, R. E., Pohland, A. E., & Page, S. W. (1995). Chemical Studies of Phytoestrogens and Related Compounds in Dietary Supplements: Flax and Chaparral. Proceedings of the Society for Experimental Biology and Medicine, 208(1), 6–12. https://doi.org/10.3181/00379727-208-43824.

65. Ojagbemi A, Okekunle AP, Olowoyo P, Akpa OM, Akinyemi R, Ovbiagele B, Owolabi M. Dietary intakes of green leafy vegetables and incidence of cardiovascular diseases. Cardiovasc J Afr. 2021 Jul-Aug 23;32(4):215-223. doi: 10.5830/CVJA-2021-017. Epub 2021 Jun 10. PMID: 34128951; PMCID: PMC8756059.

66. Oxford Languages: cardioprotective definition. Available from: https://www.google.com/search?q=cardioprotective+definition&rlz=1C1GCEB_enGB894GB894&oq=cardi&aqs=chrome.0.69i59l3j69i57j0l2j69i60j69i61.2530j1j4&sourceid=chrome&ie=UTF-8&safe=active. Accessed 12. 06. 20.

67. Pinckard K, Baskin KK, Stanford KI. Effects of Exercise to Improve Cardiovascular Health. Front Cardiovasc Med. 2019 Jun 4;6:69. doi: 10.3389/fcvm.2019.00069. PMID: 31214598; PMCID: PMC6557987.

68. Pollock RL. The effect of green leafy and cruciferous vegetable intake on the incidence of cardiovascular disease: A meta-analysis. JRSM Cardiovasc Dis. 2016 Aug 1;5:2048004016661435. doi: 10.1177/2048004016661435. PMID: 27540481; PMCID: PMC4973479.

69. Poti F, Santi D, Spaggiari G, Zimetti F, Zanotti I. Polyphenol Health Effects on Cardiovascular and Neurodegenerative Disorders: A Review and Meta-

Analysis. *Int J Mol Sci.* 2019;20(2):351. Published 2019 Jan 16. doi:10.3390/ijms20020351.

70. Priyamvara A, Dey AK, Bandyopadhyay D, Katikineni V, Zaghlol R, Basyal B, Barssoum K, Amarin R, Bhatt DL, Lavie CJ. Periodontal Inflammation and the Risk of Cardiovascular Disease. Curr Atheroscler Rep. 2020 Jun 8;22(7):28. doi: 10.1007/s11883-020-00848-6. PMID: 32514778.

71. Qin, S., Huang, L., Gong, J. *et al.* Efficacy and safety of turmeric and curcumin in lowering blood lipid levels in patients with cardiovascular risk factors: a meta-analysis of randomized controlled trials. *Nutr J* **16,** 68 (2017). https://doi.org/10.1186/s12937-017-0293-y.

72. Richmond K, Williams S, Mann J, Brown R, Chisholm A. Markers of cardiovascular risk in postmenopausal women with type 2 diabetes are improved by the daily consumption of almonds or sunflower kernels: a feeding study. ISRN Nutr. 2012 Dec 19;2013:626414. doi: 10.5402/2013/626414. PMID: 24959542; PMCID: PMC4045277.

73. Ried K, Fakler P. Potential of garlic (Allium sativum) in lowering high blood pressure: mechanisms of action and clinical relevance. Integr Blood Press Control. 2014;7:71-82. Published 2014 Dec 9. doi:10.2147/IBPC.S51434

74. Ried, K., Frank, O.R., Stocks, N.P. et al. Effect of garlic on blood pressure: A systematic review and

meta-analysis. BMC Cardiovasc Disord 8, 13 (2008). https://doi.org/10.1186/1471-2261-8-13.

75. Rock CL, Flatt SW, Barkai HS, Pakiz B, Heath DD. Walnut consumption in a weight reduction intervention: effects on body weight, biological measures, blood pressure and satiety. Nutr J. 2017;16(1):76. Published 2017 Dec 4. doi:10.1186/s12937-017-0304-z.

76. Sadabadi, F., Darroudi, S., Esmaily, H. *et al.* The importance of sleep patterns in the incidence of coronary heart disease: a 6-year prospective study in Mashhad, Iran. *Sci Rep* **13**, 2903 (2023). https://doi.org/10.1038/s41598-023-29451-w.

77. Safaeiyan A, Pourghassem-Gargari B, Zarrin R, Fereidooni J, Alizadeh M. Randomized controlled trial on the effects of legumes on cardiovascular risk factors in women with abdominal obesity. ARYA Atherosclerosis. 2015 Mar;11(2):117-125. PMID: 26405440; PMCID: PMC4568196.

78. Saman Khalesi, Christopher Irwin, Matt Schubert, Flaxseed Consumption May Reduce Blood Pressure: A Systematic Review and Meta-Analysis of Controlled Trials, The Journal of Nutrition, Volume 145, Issue 4, April 2015, Pages 758–765, https://doi.org/10.3945/jn.114.205302.

79. Science Daily. (2021) One cup of leafy green vegetables a day lowers risk of heart disease. One cup of leafy green vegetables a day lowers the risk of heart disease -- ScienceDaily Accessed 14.05.2023.

80. Scorsatto M, Rosa G, Raggio Luiz R, da Rocha Pinheiro Mulder A, Junger Teodoro A, Moraes de Oliveira GM. Effect of eggplant flour (Solanum melongena associated with hypoenergetic diet on anti-oxidant status in overweight women-a randomised clinical trial. *Int J Food Sci Technol.* 2019;54:2182–2189.

81. Shiina Y, Funabashi N, Lee K, Murayama T, Nakamura K, Wakatsuki Y, Daimon M, Komuro I. Acute effect of oral flavonoid-rich dark chocolate intake on coronary circulation, as compared with non-flavonoid white chocolate, by transthoracic Doppler echocardiography in healthy adults. Int J Cardiol. 2009 Jan 24;131(3):424-9. doi: 10.1016/j.ijcard.2007.07.131. Epub 2007 Nov 28. PMID: 18045712.

82. Sorin Ursoniu, Amirhossein Sahebkar, Florina Andrica, Corina Serban, Maciej Banach. Effects of flaxseed supplements on blood pressure: A systematic review and meta-analysis of controlled clinical trial, Clinical Nutrition, Volume 35, Issue 3, 2016: 615-625. https://doi.org/10.1016/j.clnu.2015.05.012.

83. Tholstrup T. Dairy products and cardiovascular disease. Curr Opin Lipidol. 2006 Feb;17(1):1-10. doi: 10.1097/01.mol.0000199813.08602.58. PMID: 16407709.

84. Williams KJ, Tabas I, Fisher EA. How an artery heals. Circ Res. 2015;117(11):909-913. doi:10.1161/CIRCRESAHA.115.307609.

85. Wirtz PH, von Känel R. Psychological Stress, Inflammation, and Coronary Heart Disease. Curr Cardiol Rep. 2017 Sep 20;19(11):111. doi: 10.1007/s11886-017-0919-x. PMID: 28932967.

86. World Health Organization. (2022). Physical activity (who.int). Accessed 17.05.23.

87. World Health Organization. Cardiovascular disease. Available form: https://www.who.int/health-topics/cardiovascular-diseases/#tab=tab_1 Accessed 12.05.20.

88. Yarmohammadi F, Ghasemzadeh Rahbardar M, Hosseinzadeh H. Effect of eggplant (*Solanum melongena*) on the metabolic syndrome: A review. Iran J Basic Med Sci. 2021 Apr;24(4):420-427. doi: 10.22038/ijbms.2021.50276.11452. PMID: 34094022; PMCID: PMC8143715.

Index

ABOUT THE AUTHOR

Michelle Leon is a registered Public Health Nutritionist with extensive experience in the nutrition and health promotion field. Her passion for nutrition started for Michelle at a young age when she had a special interest in eating the right foods to stay healthy. Her mother suggested becoming a nutrition professional and to Michelle, it seemed like the perfect fit. Despite health challenges, Michelle successfully completed her nutrition degree at King's College London and went on to complete a Public Health master's at the University of Hertfordshire and passed with distinction.

NOTES

NOTES

NOTES